My Body,

My Health,

My Choice

By

Marjorie Roberts, RN, BSN, MSHP

Dedicated to:

Those Who Love Freedom and
Are Willing to Fight for It

Those CAMA Members
Present and Past

Those Who Had the Strength to Endure
And to Those Who Fell to Weariness

Those who Fought the Battle Before Me
Seneca Anderson
Albert & Helga Nehl
Jim & Becky Gabriel
Bill Stanton
Marie Steinmeyer

Acknowledgements

I express my immense gratitude to my family who helped me to be what I am today and tolerated me along the way.

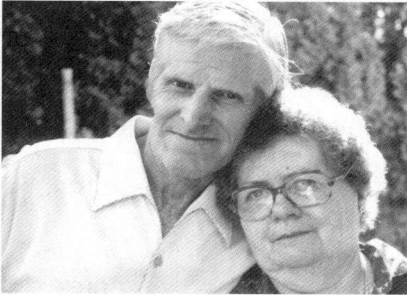

To my Mom and Dad, who gave me life, spanked my behind, and taught me many lessons of life, I thank you. Dad, as an avid reader, I hope you enjoy my first work of literature. Mom, as an angel in the spirit world, you've probably helped me write it.

A special thanks to my sister, Barb, who spent many, many, many hours editing my work. As a retired executive secretary, she served as my expert grammatical and content coach.

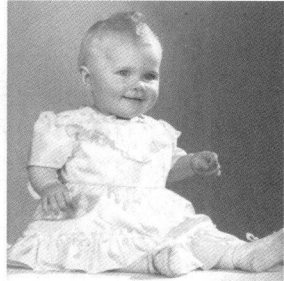

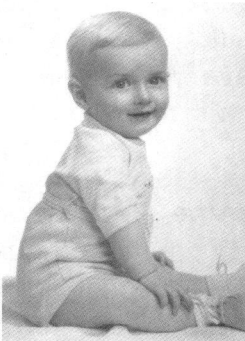

My brother Dale

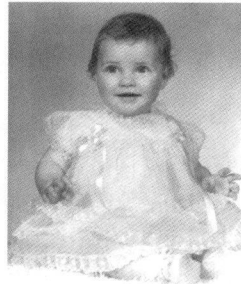

My sister June

In Defense of My Allopathic Colleagues

I understand that there will be some who, after reading this book, will accuse me of trashing allopathic medicine and all that it stands for. So let me take this initial opportunity to say, "It isn't so."

I firmly believe that there is a place for allopathy and I certainly would not want to be without it. Allopathy is literally a lifesaver in trauma, for insulin-dependent diabetics, and for many other serious diseases.

I have only two basic issues with the allopathic bureaucracy:

Allopathy is over-used and therefore exposes consumers to unnecessary toxins and death;

Allopathy has demanded a monopoly, which increases the cost and decreases the quality of healthcare, as well as depriving me and others of free choice.

I admire many practitioners of allopathic medicine and know that many of them are sincere; they truly want to do what is best for their patients. They too are often frustrated by the restrictions placed on them by their board or professional association. They have no choice but to function within this system if they want to practice as physicians. I have encountered many compassionate, competent, hard working, open-minded medical doctors. I had one growing up – Dr. Meili. I work with two on the CAMA Board - Dr. Oladele and Dr. Schuster. I have worked with many throughout my career and I expect to work with many more in the future.

Allopathy has a place in healthcare, just as the various forms of complementary~alternative medicine do. Consumers should be able to choose Allopathy as freely as they choose Traditional Chinese Medicine, Homeopathy, or any of the other forms of healthcare.

CONTENTS

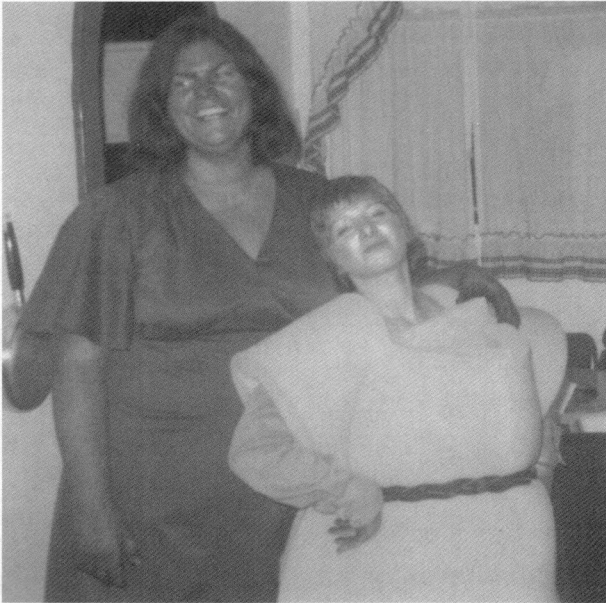

Some say I've always been a little "outside the box." Faye, a college friend, and I are ready for a night on the town for St. Patrick's Day. Visualize us dressed in green, with green body paint, and green hair.

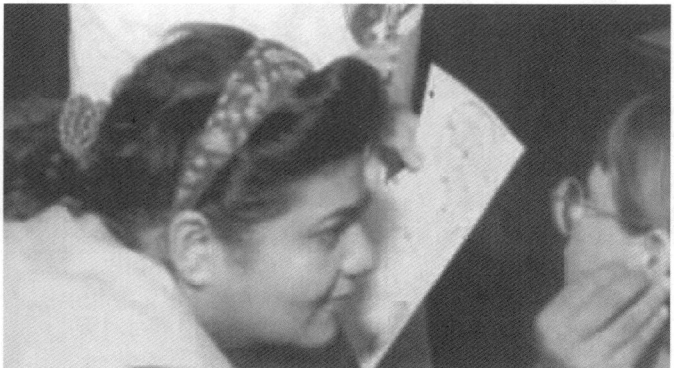

Ashu Bawa, a superb practitioner and faithful CAMA volunteer, steps out of her comfort zone to advocate for freedom of access in Georgia.

Introduction

They say that opinions are like butt holes; everybody has one. Other similarities: sometimes they stink; those of others' stink worse than yours. The differences: opinions are an acceptable topic for public discussion; opinions can change with discussion and enlightenment.

My Body, My Health, My Choice, a collection of some of my opinions, peppered with facts on which I base these opinions, is an attempt to encourage discussion, promote "thinking," and foster examination in the area of health and self-responsibility in healthcare. I would hope to recruit some to embrace my opinions but I'm sure that I will also strengthen some opposing opinions. Most of all, I challenge you to keep on open mind and scrutinize your current opinions – determine which are based on facts and which are based on emotions manipulated by others. Which opinions really make sense and which are just the "politically correct" opinions? And how do your thoughts and opinions dictate your choices and, ultimately, your health?

After being enlightened to the lack of healthcare choice in Georgia, I co-founded, along with Ron Parker, CAMA (Complementary/Alternative Medical Association) and its sister organization CAMAction. These associations deal with CAM (Complementary/Alternative Medicine) education and advocacy respectively.

Consequently many of my legislative references concerning healthcare freedom focus on Georgia – because I live here. However, the book is relevant to whichever state you may live in and has more to do with your thought processes than to the unique politics of any particular state.

Decide if you will be an individual thinker or be part of the herd. Decide if you are the one most concerned with your body, your health, and your choice. Or are those who make money off of your body and illness more concerned than you? Determine that YOU are worth the effort – to study, examine, think … and change.

Change – the only thing that stays the same - it's always present. Economist John Kenneth Galbraith said "Faced with the choice between changing one's mind and proving that there is no need to do so, almost everybody gets busy on the proof."

As you will learn reading this book, I have made adjustments in my opinions and will continue to do so. When I tried to prove that my opinion was "right," I discovered that sometimes my proof didn't hold up and I chose to change my opinion to coincide with the facts. Challenge your opinions and challenge my opinions; prove me wrong and teach me.

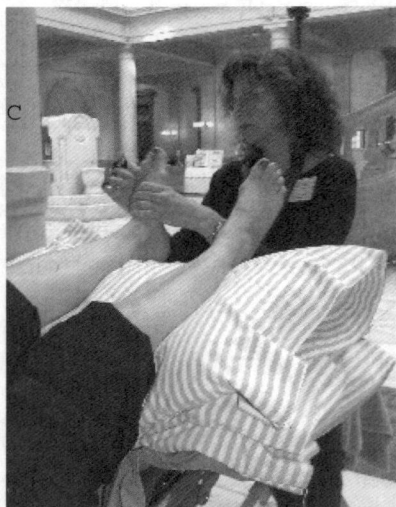

Carole Addlestone, CAMAction Board Member and Reflexologist, gives a demonstration at the Georgia State Capitol on CAM Day.

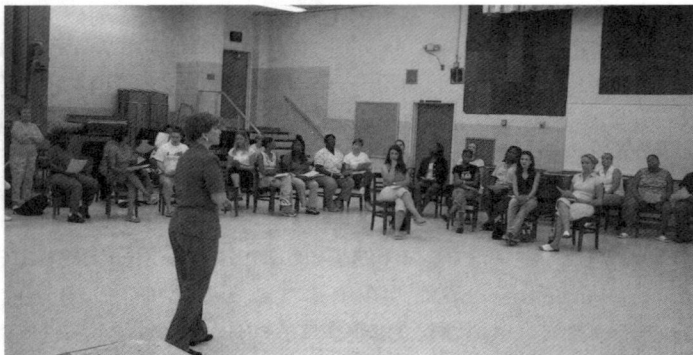

I meet with nursing students at Perimeter College in preparation for their participation in CAMAFest 2002.

Getting Here From There

About the Author

"Life is like photography ... we use the negative to develop."

Harry Cohen Baba

I know that I am not the only one who wonders and reflects and questions how events and experiences and tribulations of life put us where we are today. Events themselves - a loss of a loved one, a visit to prison, a life-threatening illness – all have a tendency to lead one to introspection, speculation, and wonder.

I am often asked how and why I continue to fight this battle to assure that consumers have access to their preferred form of healthcare, in particular Complementary/Alternative Medicine (CAM). I actually pulled out my High School Year Books, my astrological chart, and my family photo album to try and figure it out, how I got here from there, so that I might share with you.

I don't know exactly how it happened. I can only call it destiny, fate, my mission. One for which I was prepared for from birth. Just as each of you are prepared for your mission ... should you choose to accept it.

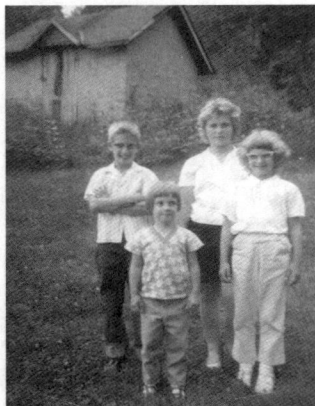

My brother Dale, my older sister Barb, my sister June, and me with the glasses. Picture taken on our farm in Wisconsin. That's a smokehouse in the back, where we smoked our ham and sausages during the winter butchering season.

For those of you who consider astrology, my birth indeed did prepare me for this destiny. My astrological reading claims: With my Sun in Sagittarius, freedom is the most precious arrow in my quiver (my work is directed towards healthcare freedom of access). My life is a quest for adventure, experience, and meaning. I have a lifelong desire to learn. I feel most comfortable with people who don't fit the social mode (alternative medicine folks?). A big part of me likes to work (my weakness is workaholism). The warrior in me is said to be peaceful, diplomatic, and consensus seeking (our inclusive freedom bill rather than turf-protective, divisive licensure bills), but one offense – willful injustice (restrictive monopoly laws) enrages me. Sounds like a pretty accurate picture of me.

I would not have considered myself a likely candidate for any kind of public exposure and scrutiny. I always considered myself rather bashful with an inferiority complex. I love the song by Mark Wills, "Don't Laugh at Me". It could have been "my song." I wore coke-bottle glasses from the age of 10. My teenage years were unkind. Wild hormones, uncontrolled with antibiotics and hormone therapy, made my face and back look like an everything-on-it pizza. On top of it all, I inherited my father's German nose, big enough to park a truck in (it's ok dad, you gave me more than enough good traits to make up for the nose) and decayed teeth from high doses of antibiotics I received for a case of pneumonia during my teeth-forming years. For a while, my not so modest derrière earned me the nickname "bubble butt."

In addition, we were dairy farmers, not city folk. This in itself was a blight on my character; we were not as "high-class" as those from town. Some of my city friends would make fun of our winter procedure to keep our house warm; we piled straw bales around the foundation of our home. Some would comment if we smelled a little bit more like a cow than a rose garden when we arrived at school.

In a society so focused on beauty and money, how could these blessings not contribute to my sense of inadequacy and self-doubt? Why would I not attempt to fade into the woodwork, give up, be a wallflower? Why did I instead work to overcome my lack of confidence? Was it because my experiences were meant to shape me into a person who could be laughed at, picked on, and yet still not be afraid to stand up and fight for what is right and just? Was it to teach me what it felt like to be the underdog, the one without the power? Was it to teach me compassion, to make me tender? Did God give me these negatives to help me develop? Just as S/He has done in your life.

I count myself fortunate that I had a mother who passed on to me her German fight, respect for the positive aspects of hard work, and willpower to persevere. My dad has on many occasions credited my mother for his success because of these positive traits. Her bulldog tenacity has manifested itself many times in my life. It is where I get my strength to take my blows, cry, and go on. It most assuredly contributes to the "how" and "why" I continue to fight in the face of injustice and seemingly overwhelming opposition.

These "blessings in disguise" taught me to know that one does not have to succumb to what is the "norm." Because the "norm" is often times no more than what the majority says it is, rather than what the truth is. It taught me that "I decide" what is important, what is truth, what is worth fighting for, what is right – for ME. And only "you decide" what is important, what is truth, what is worth fighting for, what is right – for YOU. Because my life brought me to this place, I will bring to you a part of my life – to begin your understanding and mine too. I have not yet reached full understanding and may not in this lifetime. I am still being taught.

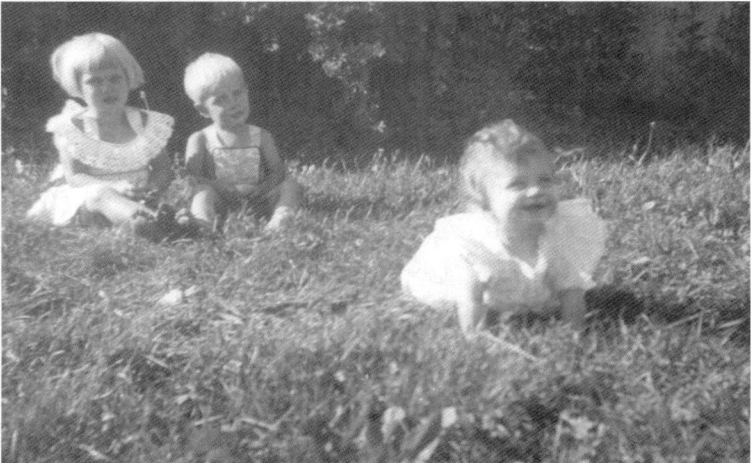

Apparently even at a young age, I had to be on the move. Perhaps it was one of the first indications that I had a tendency to chart my own course.

I grew up on a dairy farm in Wisconsin, without much opportunity for developing public speaking skills or learning the ways of the world. Since one of my daily chores was helping to milk the cows, I spent more time conversing with animals than humans. My playmates were my brother and sisters and the dog and cats. My exposure to people of diverse backgrounds and ideas from various perspectives was very limited. I was blessed not to develop preconceived ideas about people of other backgrounds at an early age. I never met a person of another nationality until I was in college. I was, and still am, the only sibling to live more than a two-hour drive away from my childhood home. I live a two-day drive away from my childhood home. Except for my brother's service in Viet Nam and my younger sister's few years of traveling around the Midwest, none have ventured far from home for an extended period of time. I never had a conversation with a Hispanic person until I moved to Texas in my 20s. I never had a relationship with a black person until I moved to Atlanta in my 30s.

My parents and most of their generation living on neighboring farms never had the opportunity to complete high school. I am the only one in my family to go to a four-year college. I believe my love for books and learning, which I inherited from my dad, my good fortune of above-average intelligence, my still-present desire to "do" rather than to simply "be," my Sagittarian workaholism, and my "middle child syndrome," all worked together to push me onward to higher education. These traits are unmistakably also part of the "why" that I continue to work for the right of the individual to self-determination. I desire to take an active role in deciding for myself the path I wish to take, especially in an area as personal as my own physical, emotional, and spiritual health. And for whatever reason, many of you have come to that same conclusion. Maybe you arrived here by way of a different life experience, but you are here never the less.

I had a few challenges in life to help develop these "fight" qualities. My first fight experience was at the young age of six when I got a "spot of pneumonia" as they called it. I vividly can call up the feelings of being examined, poked, and most traumatic of all - receiving an enema. I still remember the horrible black pills my mother tried to disguise by drowning them in jelly and the bitter drops she put in my orange juice. It was not until my adulthood that I could force myself to drink orange juice without conjuring up that "taste". But I survived and learned perseverance through the experience.

I went to a small town school, population 900, with 41 in my graduating class. I was never one of the "popular" girls, wasn't pretty enough. But my good academic grades put me a little above the bottom rung of the popularity ladder. One good thing about being in a small school is that everybody gets an opportunity to do something and be somebody, because there are only so many people to go around. During my freshman year, I noticed in my Year Book, I was a member of the Forensics Club, although I don't remember debating anyone. Nobody else must have either, because that was the last year I see mention of the club. During my Junior Year, my persistence for acceptance began to pay off. I was voted secretary of our class and was chosen by the class president as his prom date, which put me on the prom court. I joined the Dramatics Club, and became a B-Team Cheerleader (by default – the one chosen had to have back surgery and so I got her spot). My Senior Year, I made it to the A-Team (by default again – the one chosen got kicked off the team when she was caught drinking) and actually had a lead part in a play. Maybe I wanted to be someone I was not … maybe I wanted to be in the limelight … maybe it was to prepare me for being a spokesperson.

Only a handful of my classmates went on to college. My first year was all studies trying to get one of the 90 slots in the nursing school with over 500 vying for the spots. Tired of pinching pennies, I joined the Army Reserves during my Sophomore Year to help pay for my schooling, quite a drastic move for a female from rural Wisconsin in the 70s. Forget the threat of war and the stigma of a female joining the army, it sure made going to school less stressful not having to worry about how I was going to pay for my education.

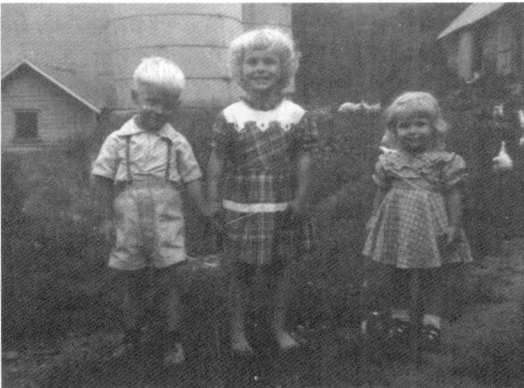

Even as a child, I had a tendancy to separate myself and be different.

My summer after high school graduation was spent working in a factory to earn money for college. Again the world of hard knocks. My parents made too much money to qualify for financial aid but my father felt I would appreciate my education more if I paid for it. So ... each of us kids received a grand total of $1000 and a calf to raise and sell to use towards our post-high school education. Didn't go far towards a four-degree college degree. I made $1.72/hr working in less than desirable conditions. I worked in two different factories, both of them in departments housed in immense heat. One was in the laundry of a knitting mill – one day the temperature went so high that the automatic sprinkler system went off. In the other factory I helped make plastic table clothes by putting large etched metal sheets covered with liquid plastic in huge ovens for them to take form. The heat affected my health of course and I lost almost all of my hair that summer and suffered scalp problems into the next year at college.

I didn't have a car so I had to ride my bicycle several miles to work each day as well. And yes, in the winter, I had to walk miles in the snow in subzero weather. I laugh today at the kids who <u>need</u> to have a car to have a job or go to school. What was once a luxury is now a necessity. Now don't think, "woe is me." You may disagree but I think I turned out okay. I know that a person is a culmination of one's experiences. Without these experiences, I would be a different person.

Another major life challenge came during my Senior Year in nursing school. I was diagnosed with severe membranous glomerularnephritis, a kidney disease. Again after prodding, biopsies, medicating, etc. they sent me home. I was told not to get any blood transfusions unless it was absolutely necessary to save my life because it would make it more difficult to find a compatible kidney for transplantation when I needed one – real optimism. It's been in remission now for over 30 years and I suspect it will remain a non-issue, no need for a kidney.

These experiences, along with an on-again, off-again, and finally broken engagement in college and widowhood at 27 have given me strength. They were experiences I evidently needed. All of these experiences taught me. I have been blessed.

So now you know. How I got here from there. My first 50 years were a great, rewarding, exciting roller coaster ride. My next 50 years promise to be even better.

Getting Here From There

About CAMA and the Freedom Movement

A Brief History

"It is important not only to have the awareness and to feel impelled to become involved, it's important that there be a forum out there to which one can relate, an organization, a movement"

Angela Davis

CAMA and the freedom movement in Georgia were birthed in early 1996. I had recently completed training in acupuncture and homeopathy and was frustrated because Georgia law did not allow me to freely help people with my new knowledge. When I first learned acupuncture and homeopathy, the intent was not to practice these arts, but simply as a learning experience and for my own healthcare. However, after I experienced the marvels of these therapies, I wanted to share them with the world. And the thought of these effective therapies being outlawed was not acceptable to me.

It started sometime in February 1996. I was out in the yard one day, playing in the dirt and watching the grass grow, two of my favorite pastimes. A yardman was cutting down a dozen or so trees to try and get some sunlight to my front door. As I was working toward this celestial sunshine, another kind of sunshine entered my life. A tall, black, lean, handsome hunk of a man who was visiting the next-door neighbor struck up a conversation with me. He was intriguing. I was immediately attracted by Ron's charm and manner. His eyes were revealing. I promptly told him his eyes were not clear and his liver was out of balance and he needed acupuncture detox. I think that's how we began the discussion on the use of acupuncture for drug, alcohol, and environmental detoxification.

I shared with him my frustration over a year's worth of jumping through hoops, at the Veterans Affairs Medical Center where I worked, trying to get permission to help people quit smoking by using acupuncture. After having a research proposal approved by the hospital Research & Development Committee and having been approved through the Human Subjects Review, I was denied the opportunity to carry out the research because administration chose to accept an outdated opinion of the Georgia Attorney General - that acupuncture is the practice of medicine. Ron was interested in the issue because of his concern for young black men being lost to drugs. He had never heard of acupuncture's use for drug addiction and wanted more information. I gave it to him. Over the next weeks, we kept in touch, conversed, and strategized.

But what really convinced Ron that we had a worthy cause was an experience with his dog.

While talking on the phone with him one day he lamented over the loss of his pet Rottwieler who had recently died of Parvo. He had taken him to the vet, who diagnosed him and then began intravenous and antibiotic treatment to no avail. Then his German Shepherd puppy began to show signs of Parvo and his vet confirmed the diagnosis and was pressuring him to either start her on antibiotics and intravenous therapy or put her to sleep. I offered to pick up the dog from the vet and treat her with homeopathy. So I did, this little limp lump of a pooch.

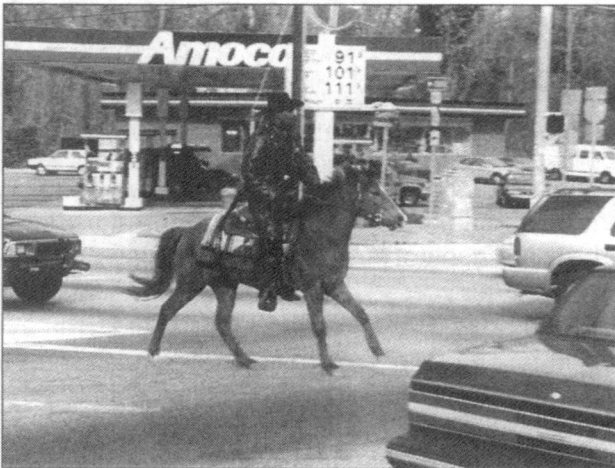

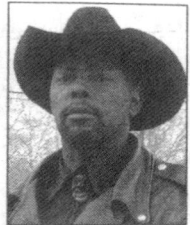

Ron Parker and his horse Cherokee Rose fit right in with traffic along Candler Road and Memorial Drive.

He thought I was a bit crazy when I had him get a stool sample from the dog and proceeded to dilute and succuss as we made this homeopathic nosode. A few doses, a few episodes of diarrhea and vomiting (detox) and my new friend was eating Tofutti out of a spoon and on her way to recovery. Ron was impressed. It made a believer out him.

There are no coincidences; our meeting was orchestrated.

In the midst of all this activity, I was confronted with a personal issue. It had started out simply as a sore shoulder, progressing to aching down my arm and eventually down my leg. I decided to have it checked out and agreed to an x-ray of my neck and shoulder. Although I had traced it back to an injury sustained when a patient had knocked me down several months prior, the medical experts tried to convince me I had bone cancer. I refused a scheduled bone scan so we'll never know for sure.

I told very few people about it, I didn't need to hear how stupid I was for not having the scan. I needed to keep things on a positive note. I took leave of absence from work and commenced a program of acupuncture, prayer, meditation, homeopathy, and bodywork. I treated myself as though I had cancer while confessing that I didn't.

This experience was a turning point in my life, refusing to believe the worst but still evaluating my life and priorities just in case they were right. I decided after much introspection that my job was killing me. When I went back to work, I requested a change to part-time status.

I tell you this because it was this episode that paved the way, freed me up, to pursue the iniative for freedom in healthcare choice. I learned that any movement in competition with the status quo is all-consuming and requires a full-time commitment. I could never have led the charge on this endeavor in Georgia with a full-time job. That said, if I had thoroughly understood the time, money, and energy that was required, there is no doubt I would not have pursued this mission. I guess that's why it was not revealed to me.

I tried to convince myself that I deserved and needed a rest from the stress I had been under. I resisted the "signs" as best I could. I tried to ignore the fact that I had "accidentally" encountered a lobbyist interested in "the cause." I wanted to overlook that he had secured a sponsor for an acupuncture bill and had talked a friend of his into providing the secretarial support for the initiative. But the clincher was when "something" prompted me to recall an old tape of a prophetic reading I had received several years prior. I finally found the tape in the back of a drawer. It discussed what was clearly the meeting of the lobbyist and the mission in front of me. I could no longer ignore and deny what I knew I must do.

One thing led to another and before I knew it, Ron, our lobbyist, had several political candidates in my living room receiving acupuncture. We were working in numerous political campaigns. We founded the Complementary/Alternative Medical Association. He had me meeting and speaking to all sorts of politicians and community leaders. I went to all types of meetings; giving presentations on acupuncture and freedom of choice in healthcare. I took my little white face to the NAACP breakfast. I road in a couple of parades, waving to the people in the name of various candidates.

Because CAMA is a non-profit organization, it could not work for any particular candidate. However, as private citizens, we could choose our candidates and go to work. Although none of the original CAMA Board members are still active, their contribution at this time was key in getting the organization started and beginning to gain support in the political community. Cindy Kilgore, Joe Orpello, and Gary Goodwin, along with a few others, worked as Joe Blow Citizen in various campaigns. We put out hundreds, yes HUNDREDS of campaign signs. Some of the candidates appreciated it and expressed their thanks; some of them didn't give a flip about our efforts after they got elected. The idea was to get to know them, develop a relationship with them. We wanted to know how they thought and we wanted them to know what was important to us.

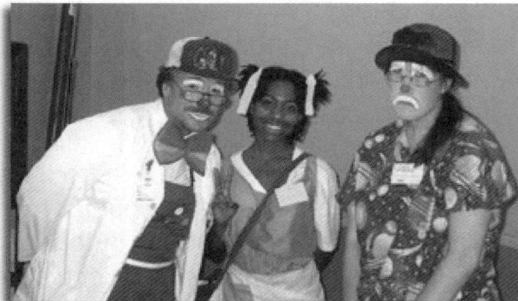

The children were entertained by Tim Morrision, our lead clown, and his team at the 2002 CAMAFest Health Expo held at Perimeter College.

I worked mostly in DeKalb County where I live because these were the candidates that could impact my quality of life. I wanted them to know me so that they would HEAR me. I had not been active in politics since the early 80s because basically I was disgusted with it all; but now I was on a mission. All it takes for evil to prevail is for good men to do nothing. So I said "I better get busy."

This intense campaign work lasted all summer until the election in November. Not a week went by without many hours invested in getting to know our politicians and letting them get to know us.

In addition, we started community educational sessions. Our lobby-ist emphasized the necessity of educating the public and policy-makers about alternative medicine and its benefits.

After the election, we had to go full-force preparing for the legislative session in January. The CAMA board, consisting of members of both allopathic and complementary/alternative medicine, had to write and re-write the acupuncture bill. We had over 14 versions before we finally settled on the one to submit. It was a licensure bill calling for a board of acupuncture. Licensure was requested because we didn't know any better, were not enlightened, had not aquainted our-selves with the public domain approach to services.

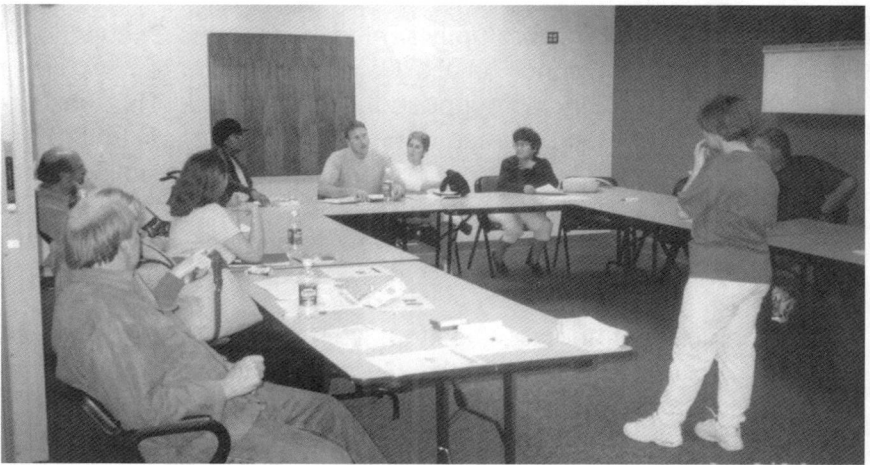

CAMA offers classes on a variety of CAM therapies as well as on health freedom issues.

Small special-interest groups hassled us throughout the development of the bill as well as after the session began. Two self-proclaimed advocates of acupuncturists in Georgia, neither one of who was an acupuncturist or healthcare provider but reportedly had financial incentives for their involvement, were a constant thorn in our side. Another small faction, jealous of our control of the situation, made threats. Others became incensed when we refused to write exclusivity into the legislation to eliminate competent practitioners to decrease the competition. Some wanted very expensive and biased restrictions on entrance into the profession; some did not want qualified people from other states to be able to practice in Georgia without first living here for a couple of years. I had almost become numb to being cursed at, hung up on, and threatened.

House Bill 145 was submitted on the second day of the legislative session in 1997 by Representataive Billy McKinney. Representative McKinney was chosen because of his long history of activism in civil rights issues. He was a black policeman at a time when they could not arrest whites, when they had to change into their uniforms down the street from the police station at the black YMCA. After being assaulted during a march, he brought suit against the Klu Klux Klan and won. We needed someone such as him who had seen some battle time and could relate to the injustice of denied access to alternative healthcare.

As expected, our bill was promptly sent to the Georgia Occupational Regulation Review Council (GORRC) for review where it would sit until summer when it would supposedly be reviewed. This was anticipated and accepted because our goal during the first half of the session was to educate and not pass a bill. Of course politics happened and they declined to review the bill that summer and the Chair of the Health & Ecology Committee would not move it forward during the 1998 segment of the session.

One of the greatest opportunities that we had was to open a CAMA Education Room as guests of the Georgia House of Representatives. Our lobbyist, Ron Parker, secured a room in the Legislative Office Building and CAMA members demonstrated acupuncture, educated the legislators and their staff on the benefits of acupuncture, and explained how it differs from allopathic medicine. Eight years later, we continue to educate in the Room. Each year we added another therapy to our list of services. We now offer education and/

or demonstrations for acupuncture, massage, reflexology, energy work, chiropractic, hypnotherapy, homeopathy, and naturopathy. Dedicated CAMA members staffed and continue to staff the Room. Faithful members such as Mike Cargile, Ashu Bawa, Kathy Mackay, Hank Sloan, R.J. Bainbridge, Laura LaRain, Darice Bossen, Jane Ann Covington, Carole Addlestone, Jim Charnitski, Avery Cotton, Cheryl Burney, Jianshe Liu, and many other volunteers too numerous to mention, have made it a success.

The first couple of weeks at the Capitol in the educational room was intense. On several occasions I heard hallway discussions among legislators and others questioning how we could be committing a felony on state government grounds. Rumor was that MAG (Medical Association of Georgia) had requested the Attorney General to have us removed. It is reported that he in turn asked the Secretary of State to remove us. The Secretary's office purportedly told MAG if they wanted us out they needed to do it themselves. MAG supposedly also demanded that Speaker Tom Murphy remove us, without success. Fortunately by then, we had Mike Raffauf, a seasoned civil rights attorney waiting in the wings ... just in case. He has since joined our Board and continues to work with us eight years later.

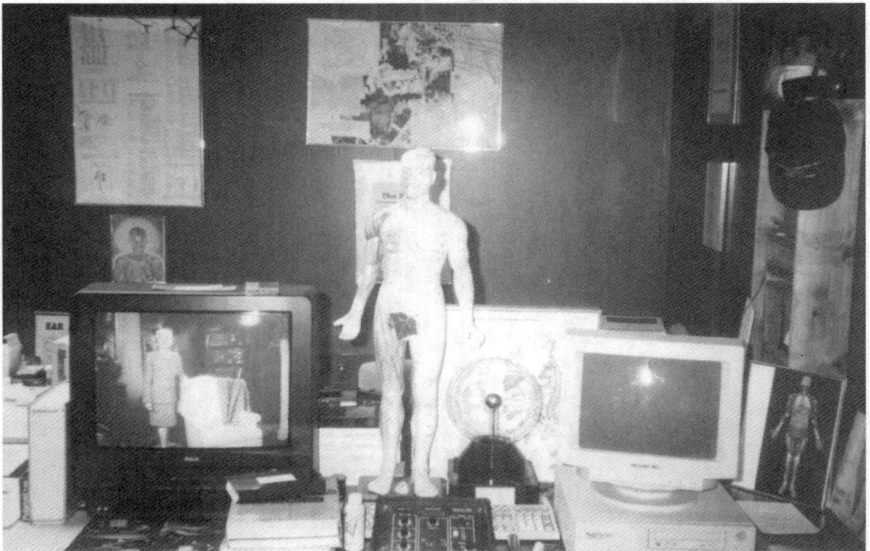

One of the table displays in our CAMA Educational Room at the State Capitol.

On many occasions during the legislative session, after working the educational room all day, CAMA members went to the Depot to mingle and politic with the legislators. The Depot is a banquet hall just a few blocks away from the Capitol where special interest groups with money put on tremendous "feeds" to show their "appreciation" to legislators and promote and educate about their issues. Sometimes the events came complete with live music and all the liquor you could drink. We attended the events whenever we could finagle an invitation so that we could get to know the legislators and let them begin to recognize us. It was overwhelming. I was so uncomfortable when we started this. I would wander from one end of the room to the other, smiling and saying "hi." Felt like an idiot. It was yet another political training session.

Another introductory encounter with the politics of politics was when we were interviewed by GPTV, the public service television station, for a short segment soon after opening up the educational room. One of MAG's lobbyists/lawyers gave a response to our comments. His response was totally inaccurate and misleading. At first I thought he was just ignorant of the facts. As time passed however, I realized he was not ignorant, just not entirely honest and definitely not to be trusted.

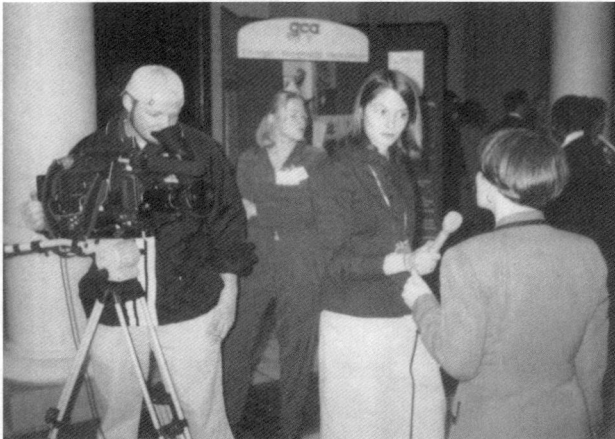

One of many GPTV interviews throughout our years at the State Capitol. This interview took place during one of our yearly CAM Days at the Capitol. We set up displays and demonstrations in the Capitol Rotunda for an Alternative Medicine Healthfair.

In late 1997, we shifted our focus to build a base of understanding CAM and concentrated on education. In late 1998, we applied for and were granted 501(c)3 status by the IRS. CAMA's focus became education. However, since this book is about freedom, I will focus on the legislative aspect of CAMA in this writing. Just know that successful advocacy can't happen without education. Our shift in focus from licensure to public domain legislation was a result of education.

Having experienced the turf-protective mentality of acupuncturists in drafting the prior legislation, and looking for a more inclusive approach, I was blessed to find Nancy Hone of the Minnesota Natural Health Coalition. This coalition was already putting in place the approach I was looking for. A visit to one of their meetings in Minnesota cinched the next move. In 1999, we introduced our progressive, inclusive freedom bill instead of the turf-protective type legislation that dominated the system. HB 749 was sponsored by Pam Bohannon, a fellow nurse and ultra conservative Republican, and co-sponsored by Billy McKinney, an ultra liberal Democrat.

Unfortunately, a small acupuncture group had the vice-chair of the Health and Ecology Committee introduce their turf-protective licensure bill. As she said "vice-chairmanship comes with its advantages" and with different rules for her, her bill didn't have to go to GORRC. After other "tricks of the trade," the bill was amended and passed in 2000; the acupuncturists were placed under the total control of the medical board. Many competent, well-trained acupuncturists are now law-breakers. The professional acupuncture association got mandatory testing and membership ($) and the medical establishment got total control ($). What more could the monopolistic opposition ask for?

Our Freedom of Access bill went nowhere.

We prepared another bill to introduce for the 2001-2002 session. At the request of MAG, we delayed introduction with the promise of working together (ha ha) to come up with joint legislation to introduce during the second half of the session. We played the game and agreed to meet with the "Complementary Medicine Task Force" of MAG during the summer of 2001. After numerous delays, we finally met several times. The participants were very nice and likable, but the bottom line was that they would accept nothing short of a

Board for the regulation of CAM practitioners, something we could not endorse. We, therefore, introduced no bill for the 2001-2002 session.

In 2003, CAMA again introduced Freedom Bill HB1040, the *State Planning for Increased Consumer Access Bill*. Representative Tommy Smith, a long-time supporter of CAM, sponsored the bill and ushered it into his committee, the State Planning and Community Affairs Committee. Ron successfully invited two other members of the committee to co-sponsor the bill and we felt our chances were good to get it out of committee onto the floor of the House. HB 1040 was introduced on the final day of the 2003 segment of the session.

Between the first and second portions of the 2003-2004 session, we formed CAMAction. With the continuing threats to freedom of access to CAM in Georgia, it became clear that a separate organization was needed to seriously counter this threat. Due to IRS restrictions as a 501(c)3, CAMA can use a very limited amount of resources on advocacy. With CAMA's emphasis on education, we needed an organization that could strictly focus on advocacy. Therefore, in April 2003 CAMA welcomed a little sister to the family. As a 501(c)4, **CAMAction** can use all its resources in promoting the cause of freedom of access.

The problem is and historically has been – many dedicated folks gave beyond their capacity but the masses sat back on their stool of do-nothing. Although we had enough support to get it out of committee, we chose not to bring it to the floor because we were unable to solicit enough support to pass it out. Once again not enough of the CAM community got involved to raise funds or communicate with their legislators. But as the eternal optimist – we had more involvment in 2004 than we did in 2003 than we did in 2002 than we did in 2001 than we did in 2000 than we did in 1999 than we did in 1998 than we did in 1997 than we did in 1996.

When you read this little book, check the status of CAM legislation posted on our Web sites for the latest, greatest news. Our educational Web site is www.camaweb.org and our advocacy Web site is www.camaction.org.

So, there you are. Here we are. For now, but not for long. By the time you read this, we will have moved from here and hope you will join us there.

Chronicle of Self-determination

A Short History of Medicine
(Author Unknown)

Doctor, I have an earache.

> *2000 B.C.   Here, eat this root.*
>
> *1000 B.C.   That root is heathen; say this prayer.*
>
> *1850 A.D.   That prayer is superstition; drink this potion.*
>
> *1940 A.D.   That potion is snake oil; swallow this pill.*
>
> *1990 A.D.   That pill is ineffective; take this biotechnologically-engineered drug.*
>
> *2000 A.D.   That drug is artificial. Here, eat this root.*

Once upon a time, in the land-of-make-believe, there were humans with strongly held beliefs who had the freedom to act on those beliefs. They made private choices without challenges from other humans. The only restraint was that their choices must not negatively impact or restrict others' choices. Only the gods and nature challenged them.

The humans determined how they would care for their health and their children's health. They decided if they would immunize their children with untested dangerous agents or use safe, homeopathic remedies instead. They decided if they would eat foods filled with toxic metals, herbicides, and insecticides or food grown by nature. They were able to choose if they would or would not eat food treated with radiation or which was genetically engineered, both with unknown dangers. Being their primary healthcare provider, they decided if they would use an allopathic practitioner (the third leading cause of death), use an alternative practitioner, treat themselves, or utilize some or all of the above. They did not fear that a visit to the practitioner of their choice would jeopardize the practitioner or themselves. Back then legislators made health care laws by reviewing facts, not by accepting the money-lined opinions of powerful special interest groups.

This once upon a time has never been.

Cave man made his own healthcare choices, except when debating with the whims of a wildcat, bear, or other overwhelming adversary. The cat may have decided the amount of meat available on any particular day and the weather may have decided the type and amount of wild foods accessible. But basically, the responsibility was the individual's.

Then it changed. Bureaucracy, government, and experts took over our decisions. The take-over was gradual and we allowed it to happen. It happened a little bit at a time. Many of us didn't notice that our freedom was gradually being taken away.

Remember the story of the frog and the pot of water? The pot was filled with cool, refreshing water and the frog was happy as could be sitting in his little lake. Then the heat was turned on, first to lukewarm, then to hot, then to boiling. Unfortunately for the frog, the heat was increased gradually and he didn't notice the change until it was too late. He was sitting in his own little world not paying attention to the world around him. He was too busy enjoying his little haven. He didn't want to be bothered with something as mundane and taxing as thinking and deciding. He was too busy enjoying himself until it was too late. He was cooked. He no longer had a choice about choice.

Regardless of how you feel about Roe vs. Wade and the sexual revolution of the seventies, I believe it was the beginning of the move towards taking back control of our bodies, our health, and our decisions. Although the movement had some negative effects, such as its contribution to the devaluing of human life and its encouragement of promiscuity, it also set the stage for positive progress toward reclaiming our freedom. It highlighted the truth that with freedom of choice comes the freedom and potential for wrong choice. It also highlighted the reality that one person's wrong choice may be another person's right choice. Who is to say who is right? Many of you reading my comments on the growing devaluation of human life think I'm wrong. Who's to say? You decide.

The environment surrounding the abortion issue, then and now, is markedly similar to the state of affairs in the provision of complementary/alternative medicine. Let me make some analogies.

Prior to the judicial ruling, the woman was viewed as a victim and the abortionist as a criminal, taking advantage of vulnerability caused by her desperation. The same is said about alternative practitioners taking advantage of desperate cancer patients by selling the patients care and giving them false hope. The practitioners are thieves, stealing their money. You've read how allopathic medicine's failure to treat chronic disease leads consumers to search for alternatives. The alternative practitioners are then accused of treating patients with worthless supplements and vitamins. The allopaths voice disapproval of homeopathic practitioners, accusing them of encouraging the patient to waste money and valuable time trying worthless alternative medicine therapy while the disease progresses. The consumer is victim; the practitioner is the opportunist. Just as the early abortionists were viewed as opportunistic criminals rather than a person providing a product that the consumer wanted, so too are alternative practitioners viewed.

A woman set on ending her pregnancy could usually find someone to accommodate her wish and, if discovered, the woman was rarely brought to trial. The provider was at risk of prosecution if discovered. The woman was a "victim." In the current complementary/alternative medicine climate, the client can usually find someone to deliver complementary/alternative medicine advice/counsel/care. The practitioner is at risk of receiving a cease and desist order or of being charged with the practice of medicine (a felony) and being forced through the court system. The consumer is a "victim."

There is a similarity in one other way but it is one you may not want to acknowledge.

When abortion was acknowledged as an accepted medical procedure, the fetus was not considered a human being. We did not have the scientific capability to recognize the fetus as the separate human being that it is. Because we didn't, it wasn't. We believed the fetus was part of the woman because we didn't have the proof to tell us otherwise. Now it is not convenient to change our belief with the changing facts so we choose to ignore the facts. It is business as usual. The same can be said about allopathic medicine and complementary/alternative medicine.

We have become so convinced of the supremacy of allopathic

medicine that when the real truth presents itself, we aren't willing to let go of the old paradigm.   We aren't willing to believe that it often doesn't work, that it is often dangerous, and that its very foundation must be questioned.   We know the facts but don't want to accept them.   We make excuses.   We want to maintain our belief that allopathic medicine has easy and quick answers to justify our rejection of promoting good health through life style changes and natural medicine.

Perhaps we will discover how homeopathy and acupuncture really work and ascertain the ever-amazing power of the mind. Will we be ready to accept the new truth?

~~~~~   And then again, our truth may change again. Years from now we may be enlightened by more facts. Perhaps it will be shown that the fetus is not a human until some point in time when the spirit/ soul enters the physical vessel. Maybe it even varies from person to person – when the spirit/soul so chooses. Perhaps we'll discover that all healing comes only through the mind. Wouldn't that be hard to bottle and sell?   ~~~~~

The next major event in the progression towards consumer rights in health care was the Patient Self-Determination Act (PSDA) of 1990. The PSDA was the first federal legislation to ensure that patients are informed of their right to accept or refuse medical care and it gave patients the right to direct their end-of-life care.   In retrospect, it seems ludicrous that we needed the court and legislators to give us the go ahead to make these very personal choices.   In Lawrence P. Ulrich's book, The Patient Self-Determination Act, he describes the operative principle in the PSDA, "A person should be free to perform whatever action he/she wishes, regardless of risks or fool- ishness as perceived by others, provided it does not impinge on the autonomy of others by intentionally harming them." This principle is gradually replacing the principle of parentalism, on which he com- ments, "One should restrict an individual's action against his/her consent in order to prevent that individual from self-harm or to se- cure for that individual a good that he/she might not otherwise achieve." Parentalism, or paternalism as I call it, supports the assumption that someone else other than the person affected knows better what is good or not good for the person.   In healthcare, the assumption is made that the patient is too ignorant to make the complex decisions required in the field of medicine. I believe that the patient may be too trusting, too hoodwinked, too misled by establishment-sanctioned misinformation, too uninformed by purposeful withholding of information. The patient is too often surrounded by folks with good intentions, who are sadly misinformed themselves, but not too ignorant. The PSDA's promotion of autonomy over paternalism was a step in the right direction. It was another step toward true self-determination.

The concept of paternalism is not dead. I get furious when I watch United Health Care's latest commercials touting "doctor-led health care." How about consumer-led health care? I really got enraged when candidate Gore bragged about fighting for doctors and nurses to make healthcare decisions. What about the person receiving and paying for the care making the decisions?

Unfortunately, the PSDA did not extend to patients the explicit right to determine what kind of care they wanted, only the right to accept or refuse what is offered. Providentially, other legislation came along to expand these basic rights.

In 1995, Representative Peter DeFazio introduced the Access to Medical Treatment Act. "This important legislation gives individuals the right to access, with the help of a licensed medical provider practicing within their scope of practice, treatments that are not FDA-approved as long as there is no evidence that the treatments themselves cause harm and the patient is fully informed of the treatments, risks, and side effects." (Alternative Therapies, January 1996, vol. 2, no. 1) Most reasonable people could not find any opposition to this Act. However, as ridiculous as it may seem to you and me, some self-appointed saviors of humanity oppose giving this amount of freedom to mere mortals.

Only deities, Master Deities (MDs) no less, should have this privilege. And only select deities, those in the bureaucracy, should make these choices. These choices are not to be made in consultation with an ordinary family physician that knows your health history, health care philosophy, and has been counseling you for years; those who sit in judgment on the Board must be the decision-makers.

The Federation of State Medical Boards formed a Special Committee on Health Care Fraud in 1995 to protect us from ourselves. Even though the Access to Medical Treatment Act includes the stipulation that only licensed medical providers be permitted to provide these treatments, it is still perceived as dangerous. The medical providers defined in this legislation are the same providers that the Medical Boards license as competent. Is it about monitoring the competency of physicians or controlling access? Recommendation number 9 of the Special Committee says it all, "The Federation of State Medical Boards should monitor federal and state legislative activities regarding heath freedom issues and develop strategies to **assure that the authority of state medical boards** is maintained" (emphasis mine). They've designated themselves the healthcare police, charged to "periodically monitor healthcare promotional materials, including random review of newspapers, periodicals, and other advertising medium."

I appreciate their concern, although I am convinced it is self-serving. I applaud their attempt to educate others about their opinions regarding fraud, but consumers should know that often times what is put forth is opinion masquerading as fact. Learn to know the difference.

In addition to federal legislation, several states have passed or are pursuing state Freedom to Medical Access legislation. As of this writing, twelve states have passed State Health Freedom laws. These State Health Freedom laws permit patients to choose unproven alternative treatments from physicians, usually for terminal or life-threatening conditions. What is remarkable is that once we are determined to be a lost cause and terminal, we can determine our healthcare. If we aren't on our deathbed, we are expected to utilize the third leading cause of death, allopathic medicine, as our unquestioned form of therapy. Wouldn't you rather have the capability to choose your form of healthcare to promote and maintain health rather than during your end-of-life experience?

In my resident state of Georgia, Senator Edwin Gochenour led the way in the passage of alternative medicine legislation. Senator Gochenour turned his misfortune of a brain tumor diagnosis into a selfless act to benefit the citizens of Georgia. After being diagnosed with an inoperable brain tumor and then researching his options, he chose an unconventional, experimental treatment as his best chance at recovery. He encountered one problem – experimental treatments were not allowed in Georgia even if the patient was deemed terminal, even if the patient wanted it after full disclosure, even if it had shown success in anecdotal studies. Senator Gochenour was forced to travel to Texas to obtain this unproven therapy for a condition that had been determined incurable. Although this medical freedom of access legislation is limited to medical doctors, and a person must have a life-threatening disease or condition to be eligible, it was a beginning.

An even greater victory for freedom of choice in healthcare was legislation passed in Minnesota and signed into law on May 11, 2000. Minnesota went to the heart of consumer self-determination in healthcare. Their Complementary and Alternative Health Care Freedom of Access Act truly put choice in the hands of consumers. Unlike the State Health Freedom laws, which apply only to medical doctors, the Minnesota Bill not only applies to those outside of the allopathic medical system, but also gives the consumer a great degree of control. Although choice is still hindered by lack of parity in insurance reimbursement and other governmental puppetry, it speaks to true autonomy, true self-determination. California and Rhode Island have since passed similar laws and several other states, including Georgia, Florida, and New York, have introduced their own Freedom of Access Bills.

The movement was provoked when during the mid-90s, Minnesota saw the prosecution of its most outspoken mercury-free dentist, its most prominent holistic medical doctor, and its most politically active and best known naturopath. In response, the Minnesota natural health community, both consumers and practitioners, united to pass

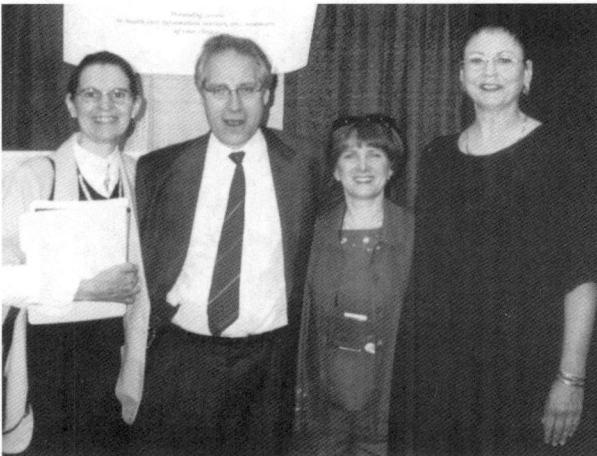

Freedom Leaders

Diane Miller
MN - Attorney

John Melnychuk
CA - Homeopath

Marge Roberts
GA - RN

Barbara York
MN - Massage
Therapist

this landmark legislation. I personally am eternally grateful for the sacrifices these pioneers made to the cause of freedom and for paving the way and setting precedence for the rest of us.

We've progressed through the "woman's right to choose" movement of the 1970s which evoked the right-to-privacy privilege, the 1980s work culminating in the passage of the Patient Self-Determination Act which protected consumers' end-of life decisions and the 1990s freedom to access movement which has resulted in passage of several state freedom bills and pending federal legislation. There has been remarkable progress over the past 30 years, but much remains to be done. Vigilance is demanded to replicate freedom legislation in all states. Vigilance is necessary to level the playing field between those using government-subsidized allopathic healthcare and those who choose to use the less expensive but pay-it-all-yourself healthcare. And, vigilance is needed to assure that freedoms once won, remain in place.

Vigilance is required, for choice is elusive.

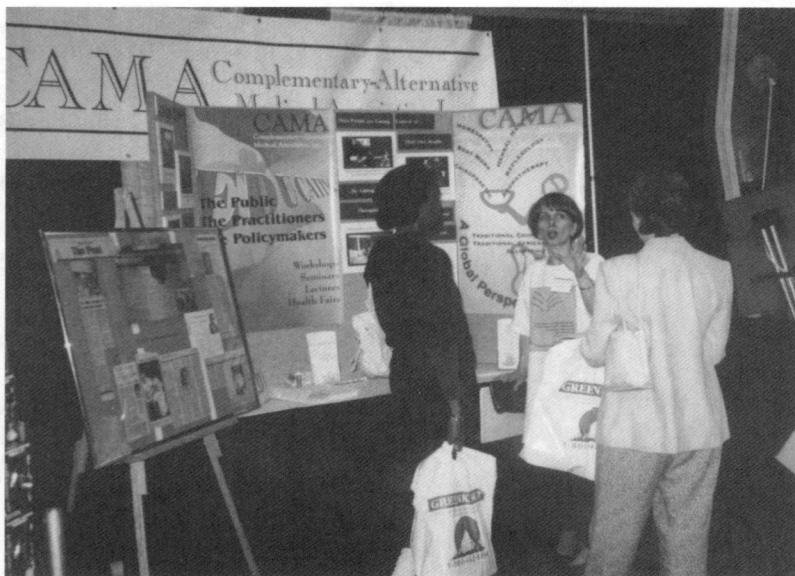

CAMA participates in community health fairs,
teaching the public about the benefits of CAM.

The Elusive Choice

"They that can give up essential liberty to purchase a little temporary safety, deserve neither liberty nor safety."

Benjamin Franklin

It's a frightening scenario. You have just been diagnosed with a life-threatening disease, the dreaded word. Cancer. The doctor delivers the diagnosis, maybe in a sensitive way, maybe in an unfeeling matter-of-fact manner. Your mind is racing a hundred miles an hour as your thoughts go to where you've been, where you want to be, what you've done, what you haven't done. You ask yourself questions: Why me? Now what? Why now?

Then it becomes more frightful. While you're still in a daze, the doctor rattles off a variety of options: radiation, chemotherapy, surgery, partial surgery. Some of these, all of these? One choice – none of these – is rarely offered as an option. Even if you're considered terminal there's usually some sort of investigational clinical trial that is offered. Perhaps the incentives from the pharmaceutical cartel are too lucrative for the doctor to ignore.

A January 26, 2003, New York Times article "Drug Sales Bring Huge Profits, and Scrutiny, to Cancer Doctors" cited a 2001 study of cancer patients in Massachusetts, conducted by a team of researchers led by Dr. Ezekiel J. Emanuel of the National Institutes of Health. The authors found that "a third of these patients received chemotherapy in the last six months of their lives, even when their cancers were considered unresponsive to chemotherapy." Another 2003 New York Times article, "AstraZeneca Pleads Guilty in Cancer Medicine Scheme" reports on a large pharmaceutical company, AstraZeneca's guilty plea to a felony charge of healthcare fraud. They agreed to pay $355 million to settle criminal and civil accusations that it engaged in a nationwide scheme to illegally market a prostate cancer drug.

Comforting reports. I could go on.

Your mind reels. You've had friends who died from cancer. You've had friends who survived cancer. Many who survived eventually died when they had a reoccurrence. The truth is, it did not reoccur. It was never gone, just hiding. Visions fill your mind. Visions of vomiting your guts out during your commode-hugging college days. If you're my age you envision a head of hair like Kojak's, if you're too young to remember Kojak, envision a baby's butt. And then the crew cut look as it re-grows - if you survive the cure. You look surprisingly like an emaciated prisoner of a concentration camp; envision Twiggy. Tubes sticking out of your natural orifices and some newly created ones. Pain. Fear. Sorrow. Worry. Anger. Confusion.

Then the real blow comes. The doctor asks YOU to decide what kind of therapy you want.

Take that as a clue. Now think. If there is an absolute, without-a-doubt correct treatment, one that they know works and is right for you, would a choice be offered? The question is not whether there is a choice but rather do you accept the selection of choices offered? Do you want to make your choices or delegate your choices to some-one else?

It used to be simple. You handed your mind, body, health, and deci-sion-making rights to the physician who made your health decisions for you. In the not too distant past, you may not have been told that you had cancer. The truth was kept from you for your own good. Perhaps it was because the practice of medicine was less compli-cated. Perhaps it was because the family doctor was just that, part of the family. He was someone who had a personal relationship with the patient. He not only cared for the patient but also cared about the patient. Today, not only is each member of the family assigned to a different doctor, but every organ of your body is as-signed to a different doctor. You go to a gynecologist, your children to a pediatrician, your husband to a doctor specializing in men's diseases. Your uterus belongs to the OB/GYN, your emotions to the psychiatrist, your headaches to the neurologist, your acne to a der-matologist, and the beat goes on. We've made a disease of child-birth, then menopause, aging, misbehaved children, junk food ad-dicted children, and now male menopause.

In days gone by, one had fewer choices, fewer drugs, fewer kinds of surgery, fewer diagnostic tests. Every day you read or see on television the news about the latest miracle drug, complete with all its side effects, a report on a cheaper or faster way to perform an unnecessary surgery, or a test to discover yet another disease, real or imagined, for which they have no real answer but many options – drugs, surgery, radiation and more drugs, surgery, radiation. Potential patients of bygone days didn't see on the evening news announcements of contradictory research studies. Now each day the ideal drug, diet, or method of treatment changes with the publication of the latest research funded by the ever-present pharmaceutical company. Historically, Physician Desk References with pages and pages of listed side effects, were not common in public libraries. Malpractice lawsuits weren't common because Master Deities did not make mistakes and we did not question their actions. The physician was seldom second-guessed; the practice of seeking a second opinion was rarely considered. We now have the Internet and the consumer can read the latest conflicting research. He doesn't have to rely on the spoon-fed version supplied by mainstream medicine. He can view health models from literally around the world.

What does this all mean for you, the consumer?

Now that it's complicated and nobody in modern medicine admits knowing the right answer, YOU get to decide. But often times you only get to choose one of the options that are pre-approved for you to choose from. Choice? Not really. Just enough involvement to make you think you have a choice, so that if it's not a positive outcome, you share the blame. It's choosing the lesser of many evils. Sometimes the good choice is available, but often that choice is withheld from you - for our own good.

It's like choosing two roads, one on either side of a mountain. You are given a choice. What you aren't told is that both roads culminate in the same destination on the other side of the mountain. It brings with it the stress of choosing without the benefit of having choices with different outcomes. Your choice is not a fully informed choice, nor do you possess a totality of decision. For example, you are given the choice between chemotherapy and radiation or chemotherapy alone. What they don't tell you is that, depending on the type of cancer, they don't expect either one to work and the side effects of either choice are assured to make you miserable. But don't bitch, after all you made the choice. So you make your choice on incomplete information, with a limitation on your choices and head out on your journey, thinking that the choice you toiled over really makes a difference. When all along the result of your choice is no more than a coin toss, with a coin that has a tail on both sides. You are the butt end of a cruel joke.

The choice to go up the mountain to the top, where the healing resides, is not offered. The people in charge of your choices don't control the road going up the mountain. They only collect a toll on the roads going around the mountain. Get the picture? And besides, going up the mountain is so much harder, you may have to change your lifestyle, give up smoking, curb your sugar addiction, exercise, or cut back on those 70-hour work weeks.

When I started my nursing education in the early 70s, nurses could not give the patient information that was not cleared by their medical doctor. If a patient was burning up with fever and asked if they had an elevated temperature, we were unable to confirm their suspicions. If a patient asked the name of a particular medication or what it was for, we dared not tell them without risk of reprimand. We were instructed to tell them to ask their physician about it. You certainly did not inform the patient of any possible side effects. It was thought that by telling the patient of possible side effects, the patient would, through the placebo effect, automatically increase the chances of their manifestation. Only medical doctors were qualified to determine what the patient should and should not know. This promoted and reinforced dependency. Patient's choices and understandings were controlled through withholding of information.

Choice can be very frightening, for with choice comes responsibility. If one is informed, absent fraud, one cannot as easily blame others for one's own wrong choices. Although it is argued that the tobacco companies committed fraud by denying the addictive nature of tobacco, one can hardly argue that most smokers were unaware of its hazards. To ignore the package warnings and other evidence was a choice, for which smokers should accept responsibility. Do we not know that fast foods are not good for us? Do we not know that a couch potato lifestyle is not good for us? Do we not know that driving under the influence is not good for us – or others? Yet, do we not make these choices every day? In these instances, we want the choices, but not responsibility for the negative results of these choices. The negative results are in the distance, and therefore less frightening and easier to ignore. Your dietary habits as a teen-ager may not show up as heart disease until middle age. It may take years for a particular medication to destroy your kidney or liver func-tion. The willingness and desire to make seemingly unpleasant choices wanes when the choices are not immediately followed by the consequences.

The advantages of relinquishing responsibility for our choices is re-inforced daily for political and societal convenience. The pressure to be politically correct takes precedence over all logic. We would never consider, nor should we, taking away a persons right to eat junk food, smoke cancer sticks, or take toxic drugs. This would not be politically correct. Yet political correctness would force me to pay for the resultant health havoc of others' bad choices in the form of higher health costs and insurance. Logic would rule that the per-son causing the increased cost would bear the burden of the in-creased cost. Choose to buy two television sets and Nintendo for the children and eat at fast food restaurants four nights a week and then tell me you can't afford to pay more for organic food. Choose to take a synthetic pharmaceutical drug and risk its side effects in-stead of muster the resolve to change your diet. Choose to put your child on Ritalin instead of attempting to control his hyperactivity through diet and discipline because it's easier and you're just too busy and tired to deal with it. Choose to protest experimentation on animals but choose to accept drug experimentation on your family as the pharmaceutical companies release drugs on the masses that have not been adequately tested.

Wouldn't it be a bitch to be held accountable for these choices? Could get expensive. Could get uncomfortable. Could get you dead.

We've created a love / hate relationship with choice. We want choice and at times we demand it. But we are scared of choice, we don't want to take responsibility for the results and are schizophrenic in its implementation. In a New York Times article by Sheryl Gay Stolberg on June 25, 2000, "The Big Decisions? They're All Yours," the schizophrenia is evident from the practitioner's perspective as well. She quotes Dr. George J. Annas, chairman of the health law de-partment at Boston University School of Public Health, "I think people have some responsibility for their own decisions. Patients should accept this as part of the price of the wonders of modern medicine." On the other hand, the same article shares the views of Carl F.

Schneider, a professor of law and internal medicine at the University of Michigan. "… doctors have become so enamored of a patient's right to choose they are abdicating their responsibilities as healers… mandatory autonomy…" he feels "…stems in part from fear of lawsuits."

There's one choice that only you can make. You must choose whether you want to make decisions concerning your healthcare or hand over your choices to someone else.

How do you decide if you want a choice? Do you want to make your own decisions about your body and your health? Do you want to relinquish your choice to someone else, and if so, how much of your power do you want to give away? All? None? Some?

How do you decide what's right for you? I believe there are four basic types of decision-makers, with variations of each. There are those who want to make decisions, for you and everyone in their path; those who want to make their own decisions and can't understand why everybody doesn't want to make their own decisions; those who don't want to make any choices and prefer others make decisions for them; and those who remain indecisive and just can't decide if they want to decide. One must realize that to be in any one group does not make one good or bad, right or wrong, smart or stupid; it makes one different. One also may jump from one group to another depending on one's current life challenges.

Some people love to declare power over others. I believe most doctors (including many alternative doctors – you can recognize them by their obsession in being called "doctor"), politicians (not statesman or public servants) and preachers (not Godly men or women) relish in this sense of power over others. It reinforces their sense of importance, their godlike status. After all, the doctor is said to hold your physical life in his hands. The preacher has your eternal life in his hands. The politician has your very livelihood in his hands.

In order to make decisions, one must be comfortable with the responsibility that comes with these decisions. Not everyone is. Not everyone wants to be. I myself am of the persuasion to make my own decisions, along with appropriate consultation. But although I'm comfortable making my own decisions, I would not want to make decisions for others. Even as the designated Durable Power of

Attorney for Healthcare for two other individuals, I sat down with these friends and only after an in-depth discussion, in which I became comfortable in their choices and beliefs, did I consent to serve in that capacity. I have a hard time understanding those who want to relinquish their rights but respect their desire. We're all at a different place.

Others rarely make decisions and actively resist such empowerment; decision-making is traumatic. These are those who choose to be victims, in degrees of course. Those who allow others to make decisions for them can always blame someone else for the outcome. Some have learned dependency and disempowerment either through societal or familial programming. They want to remain in their familiar comfort zone. Some have been burned by bad choices and have become gun shy.

They may feel they simply are not capable of decision-making because of lack of knowledge and inability to gain the knowledge in time for a safe decision. They choose to trust someone to make that decision for them – a very important decision they are still forced to make. And of course once someone else makes the decision – you still have to decide to accept that choice. So even though you think you aren't making the choice, to a limited degree you are.

And then there are those (and I know we've all been there at one time) who are indecisive and just can't decide if they want to decide. At times this is a good thing, not to rush into a decision but to think and meditate on it. It's only when indecision becomes a way of life that it becomes an albatross. A persistent lack of decision-making impedes forward movement, causes frustration, and always leaves things "hanging," never having closure. It may be better for their piece of mind and for those around them if they join the prior group and designate someone else as their decision-maker.

So unless you are comatose, it would appear that the choice is yours, whether you like it or not. It doesn't really matter if you want to make the choices.

The choice is yours ... but is it really?

Legislators - My Observations

Not all legislators are unethical; some of them are.

Being a legislator is not an easy job.

Some are into power, some are into ego, some are into wanting to make a positive contribution to society.

There are two types of legislators - politicians and public servants.

I met some wonderful people who just happen to be legislators.

I met some scoundrels who just happen to be legislators.

Legislators can't please everyone; there are usually at least two sides to every issue - they're bound to make someone angry.

Politicians focus on getting re-elected rather than on their constituents' needs.

Public Servants focus on improving the lives of their constituents and their community.

There are legislators willing to go on record in support of Freedom of Access legislation.

It is important to support public servants financially, emotionally, prayerfully, and spiritually.

It is important to support those legislators who share the philosophy of Freedom of Access.

Bad officials are elected by good citizens who do not vote.
~ George Jean Nathan

Bad officials are elected by good citizens who vote, but don't have a clue about the official's past record or philosophy.
~ Marge Roberts

Voter's don't decide issues, they decide who will decide issues.
~ George F. Will

The Choice is Yours – Maybe

*Any seeming **deception** in a statement is costly, not only in the expense of the advertising but in the detrimental effect produced upon the customer, who believes she has been misled.*

John Wanamaker

Okay, you have decided. You want to be empowered. You're ready to take on the responsibility of making your own health care decisions, not just at the end of your life but during your life. Depending on what state you live in, you may or may not have access to the type of healthcare that you determine is in your best interest, delivered by your choice of allopathic (M.D. or D.O.) or non-allopathic (homeopath, naturopath, etc.) practitioner. We aren't even talking about what may or may not be covered by your health care plan or which physicians you can use in your plan – if you are not one of the 40 million Americans who have no insurance. Should not those who are paying for their healthcare out-of-pocket be especially entitled to spend their hard-earned money as they see fit? Should they not be allowed to utilize a less costly, but equally or more effective Nurse Practitioner, Homeopath, or Naturopath for their routine healthcare?

There is a commonly held, although changing belief among legislators, the public, and especially physician groups, that allopathic physicians are the only ones capable of orchestrating anyone's healthcare. As legislation is introduced in state after state to give more choices to the consumer, the allopathic medical establishment and pharmaceutical cartel have blocked legislation in an effort to maintain limited choice and continued control. In turn, they have ushered through "consumer protection" legislation, which is truly "allopathic monopoly protection" legislation. In a Web site article adapted from <u>The Health Robbers: A Close Look at Quackery in America</u>, posted on the Quackwatch Home Page, Steve Barrett, M.D., and William Jarvis, Ph.D., profess, "Consumer protection laws have been passed to protect desperately ill people who are vulnerable. These laws simply require that products and services offered in the health marketplace be both safe and effective." If this were the case, then should not hospital errors as the 6-8th leading cause of death, adverse drug reactions in hospitalized patients as the 4-6th leading cause of death, and 12,000 deaths/year from unnecessary surgery, be cause to question the sincerity of "protect the public" rational for monopolistic laws limiting care to within this system? A recent campaign in my current state of Georgia, waged by the Medical Association of Georgia (MAG), declared that they had protected the health of Georgia citizens for 150 years. Since the 3rd leading cause of death is this protection, I'd like to look elsewhere for my protection.

Consumer choice is restricted and controlled in a number of ways. The pharmaceutical cartel/medical industry uses the media to influence, and consequently control the public in a number of subtle ways. Notice that the common disclaimer on any news story covering exercise or eating healthy, always comes with the admonishment, "before starting any diet or exercise program," consult with your doctor. As if their three hours of nutrition education, or their zero hours in physical training in medical school, prepared them to give any meaningful advice. But it re-enforces the all-knowing status of the MD in the current system, thereby influencing/controlling choice through misrepresentation of qualifications simply by virtue of position. It says "the doctor, not you, is to be in control."

The doctors are all heroes in shows like Marcus Welby, M.D., E.R., and the Medicine Woman, always saving lives with drugs and surgery, seldom preventing disease with life-style changes. It's much more exciting to patch up a shotgun wound or deal heroically with a drug addict than delve into the possibility of diet or toxic environments as causative factors in our escalating tendency toward violence and addiction. We're starting to see some evidence of alternative medicine in shows but its implementation is still orchestrated by the M.D. with the title, rather than the alternative practitioner with the gift and expertise.

A continuous bombardment of pro-allopathic commercials for drugs designed to wake you up, put you to sleep, stop your diarrhea, stop your constipation, and everything in between is the norm. You can effortlessly be conditioned to the easily digestible practice of "eat what you want; just take brand X before you eat, or brand Y after you eat." It's much harder to condition someone to pay attention to their body, "give up the pizza," or find out why it causes you problems and fix the problem, not just suppress it. It involves the four-letter word – work. It may call for discipline. These commercials are teaching people to misinterpret what their bodies are telling them. It's saying that your headache is caused by a Tylenol or aspirin deficiency, not by stress, poor diet, lack of sleep, or whatever the underlying cause may truly be. They are teaching people that there is an answer (pill) for every unpleasant experience. Is this in the best interest of the public?

All this propaganda will no doubt influence your choice, so that the choice you think is yours may be nothing but a reflection of what you have been programmed to choose.

But remember that unpopular, obsolete word – self-responsibility? All the blame cannot be placed on physicians and drug companies. Patients, influenced by the heavy advertising budget of pharmaceutical companies, often demand unnecessary medications and sometimes pressure physicians for inappropriate prescriptions. A recent article in The New York Times revealed that Merck, manufacturers of a new arthritic drug, spent $67 million dollars in four months on advertising this one drug. They expect to sell about $4 billion worth of the medication this year. Obscene amounts of money are spent on advertising drugs but the return on their investment compensates them well. A June 27, 2004, article in The New York Times, *As Doctors Write Prescriptions, Drug Company Writes Check*, reports, "most drug makers now spend twice as much marketing medicines as they do researching them."

A frightening new trend I have noticed is not only an increase in the number of television commercials for prescription drugs, but many without any indication as to what the medication is used for. It's simply "this drug is wonderful, ask your doctor for it." And some uneducated consumers, unaware of the dangers of prescription drugs, are taken in by the aggressive slick advertising and jump at the promise of a quick fix.

I have confidence that the consumer can make good choices if the consumer is given the facts and the freedom to choose. There often exists a safer, natural alternative to the more dangerous and toxic drugs. The almost non-existent dangers of homeopathy, acu-puncture, herbs, dietary changes, exercises, energy medicine, hyp-notherapy, massage, and other natural alternatives pale in comparison to the dangers of prescription or over-the-counter drugs. Informed consumers would not utilize the third leading cause of death as their form of treatment. However, the tremendous amount of money spent by drug manufacturers for advertising and the influence of the American Medical Association promoting allopathic medicine, skews the healthcare information consumers must use to make decisions.

Instead of skewed or biased health care information, consumers are often given incomplete information with which to make decisions. Research published in the December 22/29, 1999, issue of the <u>Journal of the American Medical Association</u> (JAMA) revealed that only 9% of its 3552 audio taped decisions met their definition of completeness for informed decision-making and of those involving "complex" decisions only 0.5% of these decisions were completely informed.

Consumers are making decisions with incomplete and inaccurate information. Become an informed consumer, test the facts and investigate the options.

Alicia Evans-Watts, a CAMA member who has been following the natural healthcare industry for many years, has a favorite saying, "the health care industry is a buyer-beware industry, but no one has told the buyer."

I echo her concern. BEWARE. Make sure your choice is <u>your</u> choice, not someone else's choice which you have been programmed to make.

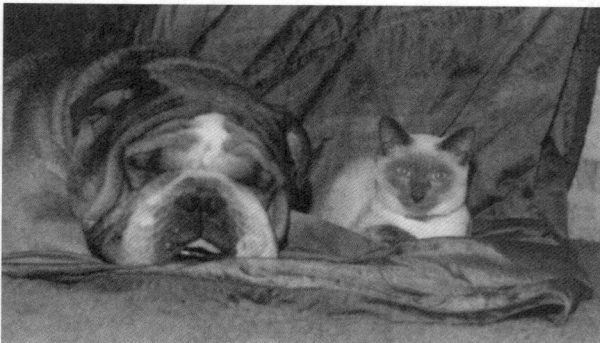

Toby (dog) and Sambo (cat) could be complacent. You don't have that luxury; you must be on guard.

Making an Informed Choice

"A man who judges a matter before he hears it is a fool."

King Solomon

Even though taking responsibility for your choices involves work, demands responsibility, and can be frightening, I believe it may be the best option for you. Yes, you may make a mistake, but so may the physician. Crossing the street is a risk. No, you haven't been to medical school. Yes, you do decide who to marry, on which career to embark, whether to have children. All can be life and death decisions, made through consultation with others with experience and/or training in these areas. You do not feel the necessity to become a marriage counselor or chaplain before you get married. You do not obtain a degree in career counseling before you feel equipped to begin a career. You can decide to have a child and be a successful parent without being a childhood teacher or expert in childhood development. You know yourself, gather the facts, and make a decision using the facts and your own life philosophy. The same opportunity for self-determination in healthcare choices can be yours if you decide to make it so. Life is full of difficult choices. Would you even consider handing over your choice of a mate to someone else? Would you consider allowing someone else to choose whether you are allowed to have a child or what sex that child should be? All acceptable practices in some cultures, but not here – the land of the free and home of the brave. But yet, you are agreeable to allow someone else, with or without your permission, decide what kind of healthcare you can receive and by whom. Have you become conditioned to someone else making your healthcare choices? Are you willing and wanting to become unconditioned? Are you willing to accept the work and responsibility that comes with choice? The choice is yours - maybe.

Erroneously, many people believe that if a practitioner is licensed, such as an allopathic (Western) physician or nurse, then the practitioner is safe and competent; only alternative practitioners must be evaluated and scrutinized. This is not true. I took my licensing exam over 30 years ago. Many surgeries, medications, and treatments, which were "standard of care" then, are no longer used. Many surgeries, medications, and treatments used today did not exist in the mid-70s. I have never in my 30+ years, worked in pediatrics, OB/GYN, or psychiatry. I do not consider myself competent in these specialties, but I am licensed and able to legally practice them. In most states, a psychiatrist with no experience in surgery can hang out a shingle as a cosmetic surgeon. Depending on the state, a medical doctor can perform acupuncture with no training or experience in acupuncture. As people become more informed, they realize that a piece of paper, a diploma, a license, or a certification does not equal competence or experience in a particular modality. The recent publicity about hospital errors as the eighth leading cause of death should convince you of this.

What can you do to help assure that you are in reliable hands? It is not easy; it requires some work. YOU should become the keeper of your health. This is the first step in assuring safety. One of the mandates that my acupuncture mentors, Ken and Kumari Wright, instilled in me was that I was never to be more concerned about my patient's health than they were. No one should be more interested in your welfare than you, not even your practitioner. You should work in a partnership with your practitioner, not hand your body over to another person. Whose body is it anyway?

When a person acknowledges responsibility for something, there is a tendency to take it more seriously and to study the issue. Study yourself. No one has lived with the subtleties of your body longer than you have. Sister Joel, one of my nursing school instructors, always admonished us to listen to our patients. She said "they've lived with their body a lot longer than you ever will and they know things about it that you will never know." You, better than anyone, can "feel" when you are out of balance. Don't let your "feelings" be discounted simply because your tests are negative or your practitioner says "it's in your head." Pursue and study. You have only one patient to study and know and concentrate on; a practitioner has many. Pay attention to your body, its symptoms, its responses, and its sensitivities.

Study your disease or imbalance. What is known about the cause, from both the allopathic and alternative point of view? Learn about how the diagnosis is made, what are the treatments, the usual as well as the unique uncommon approaches. Read the latest research, not just the allopathic research from "accepted" medical journals, but anecdotal and case studies from alternative sources as well. Study the medications, herbs, supplements, or homeopathics usually recommended for the particular problem. What are the least toxic treatments with the fewest side effects? This information is readily available to you through the Internet or public library. Attend lectures in the community, such as those offered by CAM educational associations in your state, your neighborhood health food store, or your community hospitals/clinics.

Study the different types of practitioners. What are the strengths and weaknesses of each discipline? In what diseases or imbalances are these particular practitioners effective? Do they consider the whole person, the whole picture? Are they complete in themselves or do they best contribute as a complement. For instance, you may utilize allopathic services in a complementary role for diagnostic tests but obtain your primary health care from an alternative practitioner such as a Naturopath or Homeopath. You may supplement with perhaps yet another alternative practitioner such as a Massage Therapist. Before considering surgery or drug therapy, ask about less invasive or less dangerous options and get a second opinion. Before consenting to diagnostic testing, especially invasive procedures, ask about its risks and how the information gained by the diagnostic test will benefit you in guiding the decision-making or change the treatment plan. Make sure there's a good reason to subject your body and pocket book to the procedure. "Don't worry, your insurance will cover it" is not a good reason.

Armed with this knowledge, you can become a more discerning consumer of healthcare. When choosing a practitioner, ask a lot of questions. Many practitioners, both allopathic and alternative, offer a free "get to know the doctor" visit. Don't be bashful; it's your life and health you are considering. If the practitioner depicts an "I'm the doctor, you're the patient. Do as I say and don't ask questions" posture, find another practitioner. Ask friends or a trusted practitioner for referrals of practitioners who have experience and success with your health issue. Keep in mind, however, that many practitioners will simply refer you to a friend or golfing partner and have no knowledge of their actual competency. Ask the potential practitioner for references, both from satisfied and unsatisfied clients. Ask about their success, their prices, their personality, their philosophy of health and healing. Become a partner with your practitioner and <u>not</u> a silent partner.

Beware of titles/certifications/affiliations/licensure; they can be very impressive yet deceptive. Ask what titles mean and what was required to earn the title. A certification or diploma may mean they attended a weekend course or they attended months of in-depth training. You may have seen an alarming television documentary on medical doctors who had no prior surgery experience but after a weekend course, hung their shingles out as cosmetic surgeons with devastating consequences for their clients. A license doesn't mean a person is qualified/trained/competent to perform a particular treatment, even though the law may allow him to do so.

Beware of misrepresentation of titles. I once witnessed a person testify before a legislative committee that she was an acupuncturist and licensed in Arizona, giving the impression that she was licensed to practice acupuncture. By the letter of the law, she told the truth. I knew, however, that at that time, Arizona had no licensing for acupuncture. She possessed an Arizona business license. I have observed non-MD practitioners call themselves doctor without making it clear that they are not medical doctors. Not only is this illegal but it is deceptive. Do not trust a practitioner if they begin a relationship with deception. Certificates can be made on the computer or bought over the Internet. Membership in a professional association may mean nothing more than that the person has paid his dues.

Has their training equipped them to think and analyze or just memorize and regurgitate facts/treatments/protocols? Are they thinkers or do they just follow a path because it's the accepted path of least resistance? Although professional schools are known to lobby for practice standards requiring longer and more expensive training, one doesn't need to be educated in an Ivy League classroom to become a first-class practitioner. Likewise, a long expensive training does not automatically assure a first-class practitioner. Progressive educators are developing good training available via the Internet. It used to be called correspondence school, now it's called college on the World Wide Web or distance learning. It makes education more affordable for some and increases its availability. Although much training for an independent learner/thinker can be done via computer or textbook, clinical experience is essential. I believe that apprenticeships with an excellent, experienced practitioner far exceed many classroom experiences consisting of memorization, which often don't develop critical thinking skills. I'd rather receive my care from a person who studied with a Master for one year than a person who trained in a mediocre school for four years.

During my first six months as a nurse I learned as much as I did in the preceding four years of college. Although fellow nurses and physicians were invaluable, patients were my greatest teachers. And experience is priceless. Ask how long your practitioner has been in practice. Ask how much experience they have had with your condition. Ask whom they refer to if they aren't making progress with a patient. Ask whom they collaborate with. Ask about the success rate for their kind of therapy with your condition. Have they had experience with real people or with textbooks? I can guarantee you that if someone asks me, a 30-year experienced nurse about child care, I refer them to a mother with several kids, who often times knows much more than me about a child's health care needs. They surely have more experience in this area than me, who has never had children nor worked in pediatrics.

Finally … listen to your body. If you're uncomfortable with a practitioner or a therapy, there's a reason. Find out what it is. Remember, your health and healthcare is your responsibility.

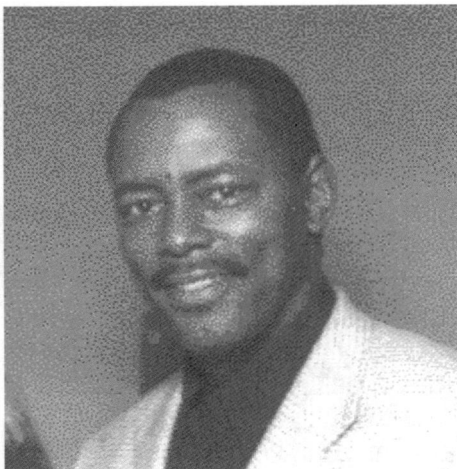

Ron Parker

Founding Father of
CAMA

Lobbyist

Political Mentor

Community Activist

Chemical Formulator

This author would like to personally recognize Ron Parker for his unwavering support and encouragement during CAMA's inception, development, and continuing work. He was there from day one and continues, at this writing, eight years later, working for healthcare freedom in Georgia. I thank him for his belief in me and the work that we have begun. Without him, this book would not exist, CAMA would not exist, CAMAction would not exist, and perhaps the Freedom of Access movement would not exist.

Ron works diligently and tirelessly during the legislative sessions at the Georgia State Capitol and out in the field during campaign seasons. He is there to "bounce ideas off of," to help when nobody else "has the time," and to be forever out in the community promoting CAMA and CAM. He has "kept me going" when I wanted to quit.

I thank him on behalf of all CAMA members, supporters of CAM, lovers of healthcare freedom, and those who will join our ranks in the future.

But What if I Make a Mistake –
the Fear Factor

"The future is not some place we are going to, but one we are creating. The paths are not to be found, but made, and the activity of making them changes both the maker and the destination."

John Schaar

Coming to grips with our immortality and accepting the fact that we have something to do with it can be a complex process fraught with doubt and fear. The pain of immortality slapped me in the face in 1979, when I became a widow at the age of 27. I had been married for less than four years to a man 18 years my senior. We were an unlikely couple. He was the love of my life. He picked me up at a bus stop and after a three-month whirlwind romance, we were married by a justice of the peace. Several months later we rode our motorcycle from Texas to South Dakota and then on to Wisconsin for a church wedding. During our four-year marriage, we did not spend one night apart. We were inseparable, until the night of his death. He should not have died so young and yet he knew he would, a confirmation of the mind – body – spirit connection.

Six months before his death, his left arm and hand became numb. As a nurse, I knew it could signal serious heart problems, especially considering his type A workaholic personality. After much cajoling and insisting, he finally went to the doctor to be checked. I'll never forget the day he came home with the great report, a misdiagnosis that would prove fatal. "'No problem – it's a pinched nerve in my back, they gave me some Valium." So I asked, "your EKG was OK;" answer, "they didn't do one." Did they draw blood for your cardiac enzymes, "no." I tried to get him back to the doctor but he was convinced and wanted to believe the doctor's report. I still feel a tinge of guilt for not trying harder; perhaps the outcome would have been different. I know that today I would have been less trusting of the doctor's diagnosis and more certain of my gut feeling. I guess maybe I too wanted to believe and I certainly had more faith in the healthcare system, much more than I do now after working in the field for 30 years.

It was about six months later. It was a Friday night, his night out with the boys. Saturdays were reserved for us. Before he left to meet his friends, we were kidding around; he was chasing me around the house and up and down the stairs. He caught me at the bottom of the stairs. As I playfully pounded him about the shoulders and back, his words are still with me, over 20 years later, "you better not be mean to me because I might die tonight and then how would you feel?" After we finished "playing," he went out with the guys and I went to bed. At about 3 A.M. the phone rang; I turned over in bed and noticed he was not there. I immediately knew dread. It was the hospital; he was dead. As was their policy, they didn't tell me over the phone but only told me he had had a heart attack, was in the hospital, and was having trouble breathing. I went next door to my wonderful friend and neighbor Kathy who took me to the hospital to find him already wrapped in the shroud. I made them unwrap him; I needed to see him for it to become reality. I now understood the term "broken heart." Interesting in that I remember them trying to get me to take a Valium to calm me down in my hysteria, I guess maybe it was their "drug of choice" that season. Fortunately, I refused; I didn't need to add the problem of drug addiction to my broken heart.

An autopsy revealed that he had suffered a "silent" heart attack about six months prior. Located in an area of his heart that would have been diagnosed with the EKG he didn't have.

I guess this was an instance when the consumer had a more accurate diagnosis than the doctor.

In 1996, I began experiencing tingling and a numb aching down my left arm. Acupuncture and massage helped but it would only relieve it temporarily. I finally broke down and had an x-ray just to see if it showed any structural damage. A patient had knocked me down about four months prior and I thought there perhaps was a connection. As a patient on the substance abuse unit was coming around the corner at a full run, he plowed into me, causing me to go flying down the hall until I came crashing down on my left side, hitting my left elbow, shoulder, and side of my head. Some of those on the substance abuse unit are often young and in good physical shape during the early days of their abuse. Unfortunately for me, this guy was built like a linebacker. Patients are only allowed 10 minutes to leave the unit and satisfy their tobacco addiction. He didn't want to miss the elevator, so anything or anyone in his way when he heard the elevator bell was not a major concern for him. At the time I didn't think much of it; I brushed myself off, filled out the paperwork, and went back to work.

A few days after I succumbed to the radiology department, I arrived home to find a message on my answering machine informing me that my x-rays were very suspicious of bone cancer, according to an orthopedic specialist. I was scheduled for a bone scan at 8:30 the next morning. I promptly called the Nurse Practitioner who left the message and told her to cancel the bone scan. I refused to accept that I had bone cancer and was not going to subject myself to the potential hazards of a bone scan. The next day, I made an attempt to discuss the situation with the orthopedic physician assistant, requesting that he examine me as a diagnostic instead of sending me directly to an invasive procedure. He refused to do any exam until I completed the bone scan. It's called "I'm the doctor, you're the patient. I know what's best for you better than you do." I refused to cooperate. My chart says, "she understands that her action is against medical advice." They had my x-rays reviewed by an Emory "expert" who personally called to convince me to have the bone scan. Both my original physician and the Emory expert "strongly recommended a bone scan." I believe they were genuinely concerned. They were sincere, but sincerely wrong.

I knew that if I did have bone cancer, allopathic medicine had nothing to offer me and I told them so. I continued to utilize acupuncture, massage, homeopathics, and other alternative medicine modalities. I professed that I did not have cancer, but took a leave of absence from work to treat myself as if I did – just in case. I was blessed with a compassionate and supportive boss. She gave me four weeks off duty to pursue alternative therapies - just in case. I wish she had done the same for herself. She died a few short years later of liver cancer. I continued with my alternative therapy, took naps, tried to do everything I could think of to improve my immune system. My massage therapy by Hank Sloan and my acupuncture, homeopathy, and other therapies by Joe Orpello were immensely helpful. My symptoms improved. I re-evaluated my life, something I had done when my husband had died. Something that was long overdue, since my workaholic tendency had again gotten out of control. I went back to work with a request to work part-time. My boss accommodated. My years of faithful service as a workaholic served me well; I had gained the respect of my employer, who rewarded me with what I needed. Although the therapy relieved much of my arm discomfort, it would still come back occasionally and more frequently after I returned to work. I went back to the Nurse Practitioner. I asked and she gave me a referral to the rehabilitation department. I was still convinced that my difficulty was connected to my fall injury, now almost a year ago. I felt I needed some arm exercises to facilitate my healing, but not having experience in rehabilitation, I did not know the exercises to do. The rehabilitation doctor spent about 10 minutes examining me and felt it was very obvious that it was related to the fall. He sent me to occupational therapy, with heat packs and exercises things improved. But again the benefits didn't "stick" unless I did the exercises every single morning. That meant a four am rollout, not my idea of an acceptable solution. Then I met Avery Cotton, another alternative practitioner, who specializes in myofascial release therapy. The myofascial release therapy consistently relieves my arm discomfort when I faithfully utilize it on an intermittent basis. I now need treatment only once or twice a year. And there's none better than Avery.

As I write this book, it's almost eight years later. No evidence of cancer. I probably never had it, a misreading of my x-ray. Or I had it and was cured by alternative medicine – an even more frightening scenario for allopathic medicine.

I guess this too was an instance when the consumer had a more accurate diagnosis than the doctor.

And let me tell you about my sister Barb's experience.

In March 1993 as she bent over to open a file cabinet, a searing pain shot through her lower back. The result was one of several emergency trips to the doctor, for subsequent drugging and orders for mandatory bedrest.

After reoccurances in April, May, and June, numerous x-rays, an MRI, chiropractic treatments, and physical therapy consultations, she decided to take matters into her own hands.

She laid out a calendar, marked the start of each knot and the duration; the knot was somehow related to the menstrual cycle. It seemed that shortly after ovulation, the knot was present; after menstruation, the knot was drugged away (or went away on its own - just coincided with the drug). She shared HER diagnosis with Dr. O. who after additional exams, discovered fibroids on the outside wall of the uterus. At/during/after ovulation, the uterus swells, and her fibroids placed pressure on her back nerves, causing the pain.

And so a hysterectomy was scheduled. Her doctor recommended Dr. B for the surgery and although she didn't like him, she had no reason to question his competency, so proceeded.

She went into surgery on July 19. The surgery lasted more than twice as long as anticipated.

After waking up in extreme pain, she was given pain medication that she was allergic to, even though it was noted on her chart.

Two days later she was told that if she ate her lunch, she would be allowed to go home. She ate her lunch and went home. Upon her arrival home - she threw up and continued to throw up - every four hours, 24 hours a day for the next seven days. She saw Dr. B three or four times during that week. According to him, everything was fine, she just needed to "get those bowels moving." Each time something else was prescribed for one end or the other, or both, to "get those bowels moving." Nothing worked; the bowels did not move.

Finally, too weak to protest, 20 pounds lighter, and exhausted from throwing up bile for seven days, her husband took her to the emergency room. She was severely dehydrated, found to have a bowel obstruction, and after numerous tests it was determined that she needed surgery. Evidently a stitch from the prior surgery had given way and the intestines were protruding through the muscle wall. This was like taking a garden hose and folding it in half; nothing really goes through it any longer. While she was gaining strength to endure the next surgery, she continued to experience the dangers of modern medicine.

In preparation for surgery, she continued to have a drainage tube through her nose into her stomach which was meant to drain the contents, keeping her stomach empty. An ill-trained nurse decided to block the air vent in the tube rather than keep it open and draining - even though my sister tried to explain to her how to clear the tube (from watching other nurses do it). Instead of listening, the nurse blew up and asked if they were trying to tell her how to do her job. She tried to explain to her that if the tube became blocked, she would throw up. The nurse insisted that it was impossible to throw up while the tube was in. I'll give you one guess as to how long it took before she threw up all over.

After three days in the hospital, she was determined strong enough for her second surgery and recovered without problems.

The experience changed her life. She has lost faith in doctors and warns every one to avoid surgery at all costs. And if surgery is absolutely necessary, she urges you to have someone with you 24/7 to protect your interests.

These three examples are from my family, but as a nurse I can tell you many, many more stories of how mere mortal consumers have more astute judgement than trained "professionals." You are not perfect and neither are doctors; don't make them into something they aren't.

We fear that which we do not know or understand. But do not sell yourself short on common sense and human judgement.

You may be afraid to make a healthcare decision. After all, you aren't trained in medicine. You may make a mistake. Well, as you see and know, so do physicians. A USA Today article by Tim Friend reported on a study that revealed a 2.57-fold increase in deaths caused by prescription drug errors from 1983 to 1993, among out-patients an 8.48-fold increase. According to a May 29, 2001, article in The New York Times, in 1999 the National Academy of Science estimated that 44,000 to 98,000 Americans died each year as a result of medical errors.

So yes, you may make a mistake – and your doctor may also make a mistake. Your best chance is for you to work together; both be informed, both be on guard, both take responsibility.

Thinking – A Lost Art

"What luck for Rulers that men do not think."

Adolf Hitler

One way to decrease the risk of making a mistake – in your medical decisions as well as other life choices - is to think before you act.

I've always been a thinker and driving the tractor during haymaking season gave me the perfect opportunity to develop this skill. Some may call it daydreaming. But like Napoleon Hill, I believe a thought is a thing and a thought must precede its manifestation. I've been told that I have an analytical mind. I think outside of the box. I think in the abstract. I believe that my many hours driving up and down the hayfields and cornfields on our Wisconsin dairy farm helped me appreciate the power of free thought, unencumbered by other's opinions and absolutes. Our amount of time watching TV was limited. Therefore, fantasy and ideas weren't spoon-fed to us; we had to construct them with our own imagination. The habit of thinking, I have found, is not a universal trait. Its cultivation appears to be a lost art in many schools, family units, and places of business.

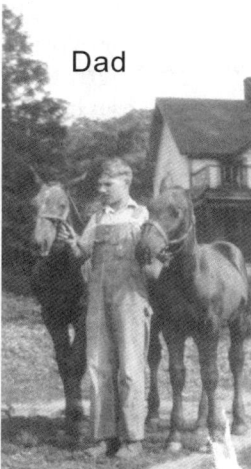

Dad

Growing up on a small family farm, away from the hustle and bustle of city life, leaves time for thinking. Nature and hard physical work have a way of clearing and renewing the mind.

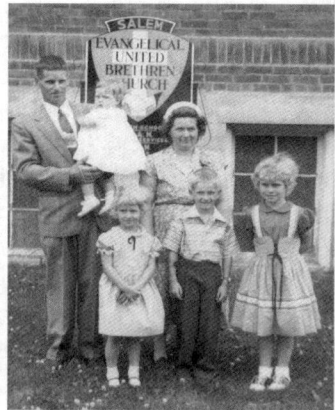

Mom, dad, siblings, and me.

It's amazing to me that many opinions have no thought behind them, but are only a parroting of what someone else has said or what the popular consensus is. No one is immune. I have been there many times myself. And on occasion still visit the land of the unthinking. There was a time in my life when I was part of a cult-like church. I learned from the experience and vowed not to repeat it. Some of my friends that were there with me are still there, much to my chagrin. For several years I regurgitated the preacher and ignored my intelligence and my good sense to develop my own opinions. My shallow thought was that he knew better than me; he was an expert after all. He went to a respected seminary, was ordained, and heard from God, so certainly he knew more than me. It was a great lesson for me. So-called experts are not necessarily expert, or honest, or always right, or consistent with your philosophy. They have an opinion, just like you and me. Sometimes based on facts, sometimes a set of facts different than another set of facts. And sometimes facts don't count. Recognize the opinions of others, but don't count them as your opinion. Think. Use a variety of opinions to formulate your opinion. Think. Use your gut, your intuition, your philosophy, your own set of facts and truth to determine your path. Think for yourself.

We are all susceptible to improperly utilizing thought throughout our life. We all act without thinking at times, when spontaneity takes over and common sense takes a hike. I think we have all asked ourselves, after a particularly bad decision, "what **was** I thinking?" We weren't thinking; emotions made the decisions. This is what advertisers and shysters count on. Why else would a TV commercial cause you to take a drug after telling you that it may cause you to have incontinent unannounced diarrhea in your drawers? Why else would you spend $2000 for Christmas presents when you can barely make your monthly credit card minimum payments? Would you think that perhaps a drug that is too dangerous for a pregnant woman to handle might also be too dangerous for a male to take simply to prevent hair loss? And you cannot convince me that the new Braun shaver and holder is not designed to look like a penis in active ejaculation. Beauty sells, sex sells, fear sells, suffering sells; all tap into your emotions.

As we work at the Capitol for freedom of choice in healthcare, we are constantly counseled, "Speak to the legislators' emotions, not to the facts." "Laws aren't made on logic, they're made on emotions." Power and control are two of these powerful emotions, which clearly emanate in the form of money in the world of politics. Does this mean it is recognized that legislators don't think or make their decisions on facts? Think about it. I believe some do but many don't. I've had in-depth conversations with many who are indeed "thinking" leaders. But obviously, sometimes logic is thrown out the window when emotions (or money) come through the door. Slick lobbyists, who know how to manipulate lawmakers' emotions, feeding them only the research that proves their case, often sway legislators. The lobbyists know that the legislators often don't have time to thoroughly research the hundreds of bills that are pushed their way. They don't have time to think before they act.

An equally dangerous situation occurs when the policy makers think, but of their best interest rather than the best interest of their constituents. Adolph Hitler said, "What luck for Rulers that men do not think." As long as you can keep the public as unthinking zombies, you can have your way. Laws can be passed to restrict your freedom, direct your life, control your choices. And those lucky rulers can do as they please, certainly not accountable to you – because you're too busy to think. After all, isn't that what you vote the politicians in for – to think for you. That way, you can blame the crooked, self-serving politicians instead of looking at the real culprit in the mirror. And isn't that what you're paying the doctors for – to think for you. That way, you can blame them for a misdiagnosis or a selection of the wrong treatment or medication.

A tendency towards blaming something or someone outside ourselves (the devil made me do it, it's my parent's fault, it's genetic) is prevalent. As I said, the tobacco companies should be held responsible for deceptive advertising and denial of the addictive quality of tobacco products, but don't tell me that we weren't aware of its dangers. The settlement reinforces the prevailing idea that someone else is supposed to be thinking and acting for us, leaving us as helpless victims. Its dangers have been written on every pack for years. We chose whether to believe, not believe, or believe and ignore. We can blame whoever we want to, but who ever makes the decision to smoke is the one to blame. When we need an excuse – any excuse will do.

Thinking is work; let someone else do it. Are we a lazy society? Has thinking become a lost art?

Say it isn't so.

I'm grateful that I learned to do my own thinking during those long haymaking days on the farm. Perhaps you have too. I don't always apply it and have been a fool more than once. And I'm sure I will be again. I sometimes put my mouth in motion before I put my thought process into action. I get upset with myself and hopefully learn for the next time. I hope you will take your responsibility to think seriously. You can not take control of your life or your healthcare choices unless you are willing to think.

Decisions– Based on Cents or Sense?

"If it doesn't make sense, it's politics."

Marjorie Roberts

It's my favorite saying but I hate it. As a Registered Nurse and trained predominantly in the sciences, I have a tendency to want to make sense out of things. Cause and effect – predictable results from predefined actions. Being raised on a dairy farm and close to nature, I grew up observing that consequences logically follow actions. You sow and then you reap. You don't plant corn and come up with beets. I become frustrated when 2+2 does not = 4.

I am frustrated by this phenomenon of nonsense. And although I have observed this phenomenon as rampant in the political realm, it is common in other settings as well.

The scenarios happen at work. All facts point to plan A; all players vote for plan A; all common sense supports plan A; management chooses plan B. Why? Workplace politics. It's someone's pet project. It makes someone look bad. It makes someone look good. Plan A is more fiscally and socially responsible but plan B pads the budget of the VP or the Chairman or the owner's son. Whatever – it's politics. And we all know about job promotions that have nothing to do with competence, but have everything to do with politics. To be politically correct, we need a male in the position, or a white person, or a person of a particular ethnicity. The choice is not made according to qualifications or competency; it's politics.

And you know about the jobs that are posted, but already filled. Applicants go through fake interviews, get their hopes up, sweat, pray; but the decision was made long before they filled out the first piece of paper. It was a political decision, not based on facts. It's not what you know but whom you know. Politics.

An incident during my nursing career is a good example. The department in which I was working was cut back in positions, so I was to be transferred to another department. The Director of Nursing called me in and proposed that I be given a newly created position on a nursing unit. The job was mine, designed for me, but needed to be posted, and I needed to interview for the job. I simply reasoned with her that this was not the right approach and to please find an avenue to assign me to that position without a posting that would disrespect the other applicants by having them interview for a position that was already filled. She agreed and simply "detailed" me to the position. She decided to make sense. She didn't waste management's time interviewing; she didn't waste applicants' time and energy applying for a non-existent position. We were able to start working instead of playing games. She made sense, not politics.

And politics is of course epidemic in the political arena.

One observes that a particular bill introduced in the legislature can never get on the committee schedule. It addresses an important social issue, the public is clamoring for it to be addressed. Why can't it even be heard? It doesn't make sense. And then you find out that although the public would gain financially, emotionally, and psychologically, a special interest group would lose financially. And it just so happens that the chair of the committee receives sizable contributions from that special interest group and/or is a member of that special interest group. Logic just went out the window and politics entered through the door. When legislative action doesn't seem to make sense – you might want to follow the money. There's even a Web site, www.followthemoney.org, that will enlighten you regarding how cents supercedes sense.

But it may not always be hard cash. It may be relationships, accumulating "chips" or favors, or simply a strong personal belief. Because one of his friends asks him to, a legislator could vote against a bill that makes perfect sense to everyone else. Someone could vote against legislation that makes sense in hopes of receiving future favors from an affected special interest group. A legislator who is chair of a committee could feel so strongly about an issue that even though 98% of the public may disagree with him, he feels compelled to save them from the errors of their ways by "sitting on a bill." The bill never gets to a vote.

A lawyer may sponsor legislation changing misdemeanors to felonies – I guess that would mean more clients needing an attorney. An auto dealer sponsors legislation to make Internet auto sales illegal. A wine distributor sponsors a bill making Internet wine sales illegal. A school promotes a bill that mandates certain educational requirements – a good way to help fill their classrooms. A physician legislator ushers through a bill to put the heat on alternative practitioners – a good way to eliminate or intimidate the competition.

And know that there are ways to contol competition other than outright denial to practice. Denial of insurance reimbursement is a favorite tactic. Restrictions on the number of visits or the levying of outrageous licensing fees are other tactics. Should you be forced to choose back surgery rather than acupuncture - because insurance pays for the surgery and you do not have the ability to pay out-of-pocket for an acupuncturist? Should you be allowed unlimited visits and unlimited funds to subject yourself to invasive medical care but be restricted to twelve chiropratic visits to "get it fixed?"

It make sense, to cover your ass, protect your pocketbook, to maintain control – but it's still politics.

Workplace Politics - decisions not based on what's right, but on favors and friendships.

Legislative Politics - legislation not based on what's good for the constituents, but what serves the politician.

I really get mad when non-sense politics get in the way of MY personal life, my personal choices, choices that right or wrong, good or bad, hurt no one but myself. In particular, I don't want my healthcare choices restricted by some legislator playing politics with my life. Over what area of my life should I have unequivocal choice if it is not that of my own body?

Does it make sense or is it politics that others have a greater right to determine how I treat my body than I do? No. It's politics – control and money.

Should consumers, especially those who pay out-of-pocket, be forced to go to a medical doctor when they would rather go to a Nurse Practitioner, a Homeopath, a Naturopath, or whoever? Whose body is it anyway? And in this case, whose money is it anyway?

The continuing attempt to suppress natural health care choices (inherently safe) and promote allopathic medicine (the third leading cause of death) is so nonsensical that it defies all logic. Monopoly control not only decreases quality but increases cost.

And so it has been, is, and will be. Unless you change it.

Your challenge is to recognize politics when it rears its ugly, thieving, dishonest head, and differentiate it from that which makes sense. So if it doesn't make sense – assume it's politics and begin to examine, to follow the money, to question.

It's your responsibility; it's your body, your health, and your choice.

Do You Need a Reason to Take Control?

"It makes cents to mandate one of the leading causes of death as your form of healthcare."

Marjorie Roberts

A commentary published in the July 26, 2000, issue of the <u>Journal of the American Medical Association</u> (<u>JAMA</u>) suggests that the total death toll from iatrogenic (caused by medical treatment) causes is 225,000/year, the third leading cause of death, after heart disease and cancer.

A major factor in this amazing death rate is the large number of deaths from prescription drugs. As far back as 1995, research published in the <u>Archives of Internal Medicine</u> concluded that drug-related morbidity and mortality was estimated to cost $76.6 billion in the ambulatory setting alone. And a 1995 <u>JAMA</u> article concluded, "Adverse drug events were common ..." A meta-analysis published in 1998 by <u>JAMA</u> suggests that adverse drug reactions in hospitalized patients are the **fourth to sixth leading cause of death**.

The use of medications has become so commonplace that we have become numb to the potential of their danger. <u>JAMA</u> reported in their December 10, 1997, issue, "Adverse reactions to drugs or biological agents are frequent consequences of medical treatment since few, if any, medications produce beneficial effects alone." The question is whether these adverse effects are lethal, crippling, or simply an inconvenience. Just because a drug is on the market does not mean it is safe. <u>The New York Times</u>, June 8, 2002, *U.S. Lets Drug Tied to Deaths Back on Market*, reports on Lotronex, a prescription treatment for irritable bowel syndrome. It was taken off the market, less than 10 months after it was approved, when it was linked to severe intestinal problems and several deaths. As of this writing it is prepared to go back on the market with the warning that "the new rules leave considerable responsibility with doctors, pharmacists, and patients to use it correctly and to watch for early signs of intestinal problems, which can be fatal." Hum, were they not responsible and watching for early signs of intestinal problems before?

A USA Today, March 20, 1998, article offers some alarming statistics: "32,000 elderly people suffer hip fractures yearly in falls caused by adverse drug reactions; 16,000 car accidents are attributed to such reactions; drug misuse accounts for $20 billion in hospital costs each year; 17.5% of the 30 million people on Medicare who are not in nursing homes receive drugs that are unsafe or duplicate prescriptions; more than 30% of 75-85-year-olds are prescribed contraindicated drugs." A remarkable third of 75-85-year-olds are prescribed drugs that they should not have. Aren't you really excited about expanding Medicare drug coverage? We'll have our elderly dropping like flies when the medical providers and senior citizens are given a blank check.

I think it is too late to turn back the hands of time to an era when all our health decisions were made for us and paternalistic healthcare was the norm. According to evidence presented in a recent Commentary in JAMA, July 26, 2000, 20% to 30% of patients receive contraindicated care. In addition, the author cites U.S. estimates of the "combined effect of errors and adverse effects that occur because of iatrogenic damage not associated with recognizable error include: 12,000 deaths/year from unnecessary surgery, 7,000 deaths/year from medication errors in hospitals, 20,000 deaths/year from other errors in hospitals, 80,000 deaths/year from nosocomial (hospital-acquired) infections in hospitals, and 106,000 deaths/year from non-error, adverse effects of medication."

The 2000 World Health Organization report ranked the United States 37th among 191 countries in the quality of overall health care. The past "keepers of our health" may not necessarily be the safest "keepers." Perhaps the individual with a vested interest in staying healthy and alive, an individual who knows himself better than the doctor or anyone else, someone who only has one patient to look after (not a physician who has hundreds shuffling through the office, one every 15 minutes), is the best person to make your healthcare decisions.

I would not want to be without the expertise of allopathic medicine when presented with trauma or an immediate life-threatening condition; life-saving drugs and surgery are sometimes necessary.

However, they are often used when less toxic therapies with less risk and fewer side effects would be as effective or more effective. Consumers often do not understand the risks of drugs and their potential for injury and death. Drugs are used freely and it is not uncommon for patients to be on multiple medications, further increasing the risks for potential negative interactions between drugs.

The relationships among physicians who prescribe drugs, professional journals who depend on advertising revenue from manufacturers, and pharmaceutical companies poised to make billions from the sale of these drugs cannot be ignored. The New England Journal of Medicine, a prestigious medical publication, recently admitted to violating its conflict-of-interest policy in 19 of 40 drug therapy reviews. For example, although a researcher signed a statement declaring that she had not nor would receive any monetary rewards from the pharmaceutical company for which she wrote a favorable review, she then accepted $1.7 million dollars in research funding. Pharmaceutical companies often pay physicians to speak and write in support of a drug, sometimes in the form of future research grants. In addition, pharmaceutical companies fund their own drug studies and the respective drug may be sold to the public before any independent clinical studies are done.

Unless I was absolutely sure that there was no other option, I would personally not consider using a drug until it's been on the market for at least five years and I have an idea of the body count. Numerous drugs have been approved for the market only to be recalled. Rezulin, a diabetic drug, was pulled after it was linked to 90 cases of liver failure and 63 deaths. Posicor was withdrawn from the market when it was discovered that more than 25 other drugs were potentially dangerous when used in conjunction with it. Duract was withdrawn after reports of severe liver failure resulted in four deaths and eight liver transplants. Propulsid was pulled from the market after reports of serious adverse reactions, including death. Many other drugs, such as Phen-Fen and Viagra, have been either recalled or are under re-labeling warnings because of adverse effects.

And don't be deceived when "unbiased" groups endorse drugs. They too may be influenced to speak a contaminated truth. The British Medical Journal, March 29, 2003, reports that *Us Too! International*, a lay men's group, which campaigns for men to take the prostate specific antigen screen test, gets 95% of its funding from the pharmaceutical industry. This "charitable" organization held $799,012 in net assets at the end of 2000. They further report, "a 1999 investigation by 17 states' attorney generals found that buying trust is a key goal for drug companies that sponsor non-profit groups … a strategy known as "passion branding." An October 5, 2000, <u>New York Times</u> article reported on a "consumer activist" representing three grass-roots organizations who testified for Congress that the drug stores, rather than the drug companies, were to blame for the high cost of prescription drugs. What the panel of Senators was not told was that "she also worked full-time for a public relations company whose clients include the Pharmaceutical Research and Manufacturers of America, the drug industry's trade group." And it just so happens that this same industry trade group provided seed money and public relations expertise to one of the non-profits she represented. Oh what a tangled web we weave, when we want to deceive.

And don't forget our national celebrities. *Pushing Pills with Piles of Money*, <u>The New York Times</u>, October 5, 2000, reports on former Olympic stars pushing drugs on talk shows and while speaking to private groups, never revealing that they are on the payroll of the pharmaceutical companies. You may have even noticed drugs being referred to in sitcoms and discussed on late night talk shows. A gazillion dollars can buy lots of positive reports ... and numb one's conscious.

An August 12, 2003, article in <u>The New York Times</u> reported on a hospital that "paid $54 million to the government to resolve accusations that their medical doctors conducted unnecessary heart procedures and operations on hundreds of healthy patients." Their "business model was based on maximizing the dollars it could collect from Medicare." Again, I say, aren't you really excited about expanding Medicare drug coverage? It's such a dependable system for surgery; it must be a great system for drug coverage as well. Let's make it bigger so it's even harder to monitor.

Another <u>The New York Times</u> article, *As Doctors Write Prescriptions, Drug Company Writes Check*, published June 27, 2004 reported that Pfizer agreed to pay $430 million and plead guilty to criminal charges... AstraZeneca paid $355 million last year and TAP Pharmaceuticals paid $875 million in 2001; each pleaded guilty to criminal charges.

And yet another <u>The New York Times</u> article, July 16, 2004, *Guilty Plea Seen for Drug Maker*, reports that Schering-Plough agreed to pay $350 million in fines and plead guilty to criminal charges that it cheated the Medicaid program. The article also reveals that Bayer paid $257 million and GlaxoSmithKline paid $86.7 million for similar allegations and Pfizer agreed in May to pay $430 million to settle allegations that a subsidiary marketed a drug improperly.

... A book could be written just on the recurring illegalities of the legal drug market.

I could go on and on with example after example. Suffice it to say; there are no safe drugs or procedures; pharmaceutical companies are out for your money, not your health; people, including doctors, researchers, celebrities and heroes, are vulnerable to lying for financial gain. In emergencies, drugs, procedures, and surgery may be necessary and life saving, but YOU must control when you use them, know that they are dangerous and not without risk but with almost certain damage to some degree. The nation's healthcare is out of control.

Both allopathic and CAM therapy are vital to our health and longevity, valid and needed. Just don't get the idea that either one has all the answers for all diseases or is always trustworthy and the "right" thing to do. If I get my leg caught in a steamroller – send me to an allopath to either chop it off or sew it back on WITH anesthesia. And then let me use homeopathy, acupuncture, hypnotherapy, energy work, and massage for my healing, physically, mentally, and spiritually. Let me control my person.

From The New York Times

October 29, 2002
Documents Show Effort to Promote Unproven Drug
By MELODY PETERSEN

October 1, 2002
Drug Industry Is Told to Stop Gifts to Doctors
By ROBERT PEAR

December 26, 2002
Drug Makers Battle Plan to Curb Rewards for Doctors
By ROBERT PEAR

December 4, 2002
Investigators Find Repeated Deception in Ads for Drugs
By ROBERT PEAR

June 21, 2003
AstraZeneca Pleads Guilty in Cancer Medicine Scheme
By MELODY PETERSEN

April 17, 2003
Bayer Agrees to Pay U.S. $257 Million in Drug Fraud
By MELODY PETERSEN

May 20, 2003
Doctor Admits He Did Needless Surgery on the Mentally Ill
By CLIFFORD J. LEVY

June 13, 2003
Guidant Admits That It Hid Problems of Artery Tool
By KURT EICHENWALD

August 12, 2003
How One Hospital Benefited on Questionable Operations
By KURT EICHENWALD

June 27, 2004
As Doctors Write Prescriptions, Drug Company Writes a Check
By GARDINER HARRIS

A Veil of Deception

"The power of an air force is terrific when there is nothing to oppose it. "

Winston Churchill

Webster defines "to integrate" as "to put or bring together into a whole," "to make whole or complete by adding or bringing together parts." If we were to use the term "integrative medicine" to mean that we are attempting to make healthcare complete and whole by offering the individual the option of choosing from a variety of modalities, each complete in itself and yet able to complement the other, it is certainly a good thing. If, however, we promote "integrative medicine" as a catchy phrase to make palatable the absorbing of select "alternative" medicine treatments into the allopathic model, we are doing a disservice to the public and the traditions of equally valid and legitimate healthcare models. I fear that the latter scenario is true. "Alternative Medicine" has been perceived as an outcast for so long that I believe there may be a tendency on the part of some alternative practitioners to relinquish the uniqueness and separateness of their model for the sake of acceptance into the "mainstream" via integration. Many assume, or want to believe, that the intent of the popularized term "integrative medicine" is truly the unification of all the disciplines together. However, in order to accomplish a truly integrative system, we need a level playing field. This is not the case.

One of the leaders in the "integrative medicine" movement has been the University of Arizona College of Medicine. Their Web site states "To develop a true synthesis of conventional and alternative practices, it is critical that the Program be based in an allopathic teaching institution." One of the goals of the program is listed to "Produce leaders in this new discipline of medicine who will...set policy and direction for healthcare in the 21st century." Who assigned allopathic medicine as the watchdogs and policy-setters for our future healthcare? I think that we need to look no further than our present state of healthcare to see that maybe another group needs to be "in charge." Perhaps the consumer? The Flagstaff Medical Center (FMC) says "All integrative medicine services at FMC will be physician directed."

It is clear to me that the working definition of integrative medicine is allopathic medicine with the allopathic physician remaining in charge, but utilizing on a select basis those portions of different modalities that have become popular with the public or partially accepted by his peers. For instance, some doctors utilize acupuncture, but can only accept its use for select conditions such as pain, and may discount the philosophy of Traditional Chinese Medicine (TCM) that birthed this therapy and the explanation of how it works. The term often used is "medical acupuncture" to differentiate it from the acupuncture practiced by those trained within the TCM paradigm. Even when the treatment, such as acupuncture or herbal therapy, is delivered by a non-allopathic practitioner, the person at the helm remains the allopathic physician. A few states recognize Oriental Medical Doctors, Homeopaths, and Naturopaths as primary care providers, but most state laws still reserve the position of authority to that of the allopathic physician.

The term "integrative medicine" should therefore be portrayed as it is, a sub-specialty of allopathic medicine. However, some falsely characterize integrative medicine as an equal union and respect between allopathic medicine and complementary/alternative medicine. There is much confusion already in our ever-changing health field. I believe it is important to accurately represent concepts in the spirit of truth and their "working" definition rather than trying to wrap them in more agreeable but misleading terminology.

I am encouraged that more allopathic medicine professionals are beginning to see the advantages in modalities outside the allopathic model, that there is a move among allopathic practitioners to utilize less invasive, less toxic therapies. I am delighted to see a greater emphasis on prevention, lifestyle, and patient involvement. I think it is appropriate for allopathic practitioners to become familiar with different modes of medicine and indeed integrate some of the modalities into their practice. But to absorb various health care delivery systems under the auspices of allopathic medicine and call it "integrative medicine," denies the validity of distinct and equally valuable healthcare delivery systems such as Ayevedic, Traditional Oriental Medicine, Naturopathy, Chiropractic, Traditional African Medicine, and Homeopathy. One does not get "the best of both worlds" when an allopathic doctor delivers a portion of an alternative medicine modality within the allopathic medicine model. One gets "the best of many worlds" when all disciplines work together on equal turf for the benefit of the consumer.

At one point during our Georgia negotiations, the acting Executive Director of the Medical Association of Georgia (MAG) reaffirmed that they would consider nothing short of a Board as acceptable oversight for alternative practitioners. We shared our misgivings concerning the formation of a Board - it was not needed; it would increase costs to the state, consumer, and practitioner; it would not be approved by the legislature; it would not be supported by the Georgia Occupational Regulation Review Council. Of course his response was to suggest that we consider putting alternative practitioners under the Medical Board.

Sound familiar? In Georgia, the precedent was set when acupuncturists were placed under the Board's control in 2000. They too started out with visions of their own board. CAMA unsuccessfully opposed this legislation. We were concerned that it would facilitate allopathy's plan to regulate and control all of CAM. It appears that the concern was well founded. Whether the Georgia Medical Board wants to control all of CAM or will choose those they feel would be most lucrative and eliminate/ignore the rest is an unknown. Do you even know what's happening in YOUR state? What are allopathy's plans for your state's access to CAM?

Although familiarity and some incorporation of alternative medicine into allopathic medicine is necessary to properly advise patients, treat them, or refer them to an appropriate alternative practitioner when warranted, traditional medical practices must also remain as separate healthcare models. I think it is vital that the practitioners of various health philosophies work together, refer back-and-forth, and teach each other. In this time of recognizing and celebrating diversity in the areas of culture, religion, and doctrine, it is curious that the allopathic medical model is urging just the opposite. Instead of assimilating the non-allopathic healthcare models into the allopathic model, we need to recognize and acknowledge alternatives to the allopathic model. We must remember that the United

States is not the world and 80% of the world utilizes non-allopathic medicine. We need to respect different ways of perceiving and administering health, wellness, and health care.

Since the term "integrative medicine" has come to signify a sub-specialty of allopathic medicine, I would propose the term "global medicine" be used to communicate respect for all forms of medicine. I would prefer to strive toward a vision of global medicine, of which integrative (allopathic sub-specialty) medicine is considered just one delivery method among the many throughout the world, each of equal worth. The individual will be the one to make the decision about which form to utilize for which malady, to maintain health and prevent disease, in whatever period of their life, and delivered by whom they choose. Whether we choose Ayevedic, Traditional Chinese Medicine, Naturopathy, Chiropractic, Traditional African Medicine, or Homeopathy, it should be our individual choice, based on our belief system. It is up to us to orchestrate our own healthcare from the arena of global medicines. We must decide whether and when to use them together or separately and how and when we utilize which modality. If anyone is to truly integrate medicine it needs to be us, the consumer.

Protect the Public Fallacy

"If you have ten thousand regulations you destroy all respect for the law."

Sir Winston Churchill

Former Governor Zell Miller wrote in a campaign flyer for former Governor Roy Barnes, "Decisions like choosing your own doctor and hospital should be yours and yours alone." Surely he meant to include Doctors of Chiropractic, Doctors of Homeopathy, Doctors of Oriental Medicine, Doctors of Naturopathy, Doctors of ... you get the picture.

As we have seen, our current "mainstream" health care industry is in a mess. As the third leading cause of death, it is hardly the savior of the people. In addition, a report by the National Coalition on Health Care revealed that nearly 20 percent of the non-elderly population were uninsured in early 1996, an estimated 44.5 million persons. And the federal Health Care Financing Administration released a report that "health care spending will rise from 13.6% of gross domestic product (GDP) to 16.6% of GDP over the next ten years..." This is not good news.

But what do we, as supporters and promoters of CAM learn from this? Many CAM practitioners, anxious to be "accepted" by the mainstream medical regime and desirous of insurance reimbursement, are attempting to pattern Complementary and Alternative Health Care delivery after this crumbling, inefficient, over-priced, over-regulated, discriminatory, often ineffective, model. I personally believe it unwise to pattern oneself after a system that is disintegrating. We are supposed to learn from history, to learn from past experience. As Albert Einstein said "The significant problems we have cannot be solved at the same level of thinking we were at when we created them." Let's look at and evaluate the situation. Let's develop a new paradigm, not blindly pattern ourselves after a crumbling dinosaur just because it's the current model. Even though it is outdated verbiage, "We need a paradigm shift."

Although I believe the disarray of our health care system is multi-dimensional and attributable to many factors, I want to deal with the licensure/regulation issue. The prevailing approach to regulation demands licensure, rather than the equally effective, and in some aspects superior, avenues of non-mandatory certification or registration.

One of the least restrictive forms of governmental regulation is state registration. Registration mandates only that individuals be required to list their names in some official register if they engage in certain kinds of activities. There is no provision for denying the right to engage in the activity to anyone who is willing to list his name. It does not mandate a level of training nor does it mandate that the level of training and/or experience be revealed. One of the dangers of registration is that it often leads to forced certification and then to full licensure. This was the case with acupuncture in Vermont, which for many years functioned under state registration without problems. However, special interest groups maneuvered a change mandating first certification and then licensure.

Certification allows for verification that an individual has certain skills, but may not prevent, in any way, the practice of an occupation using these skills by people who do not have such a certificate. For example, the state may authorize certified massage therapists that have taken a test or completed a designated level of education to practice and use the title certified massage therapist. This does not prevent others from practicing massage therapy; they cannot however use the title "certified."

Licensure is the most restrictive form of regulation. Like certification, licensure requires some demonstration of competence, but goes one step further and denies the right of anyone who does not have such a license to practice. Licensed professions work under specific defined scopes of practice. Therein is the problem. Professional scopes of practice are generally defined broadly. These broad definitions can be interpreted in such a way as to put many competent practitioners at risk. For example, the Official Code of Georgia (OCG) 43-26-3. (6) defines the *practice of nursing* as "to perform for compensation ... any act in the care and counsel of the ill, injured, or infirm, and in the promotion and maintenance of health with individuals, groups, or both throughout the life span ..." Could this not include almost any practitioner offering healthcare in any shape or form?

OCG 43-34-26 G states "(a) If any person shall hold himself out to the public as being engaged in the diagnosis or treatment of disease or injuries of human beings, or shall suggest, recommend, or prescribe any form of treatment for the palliation, relief, or cure of any physical or mental ailment of any person, with the intention of receiving therefor, either directly or indirectly, any fee, gift, or compensation whatsoever, or shall maintain an office for the reception, examination, or treatment of diseased or injured human beings, or shall attach the title "M.D.," "Oph.," "D.," "Dop.," "Surgeon," "Doctor," "D.O.," "Doctor of Osteopathy," either alone or in connection with other words, or any other word or abbreviation to his name indicative that he is engaged in the treatment of diseased, defective, or injured human beings, and shall not in any of these cases then possess a valid license to practice medicine under the laws of this state, he shall be deemed to be practicing medicine without complying with this chapter and shall be deemed in violation of this chapter." Should suggesting and recommending be the practice of medicine or should surgery, prescribing drugs or administering radiation be the "practice of medicine?" Which makes sense to you?

Harris Coulter asks, "Nearly all the alternative providers reject the allopathic paradigm in whole or in part, so how can they be regulated on the basis of this paradigm? ….allopathy has always been regulated on the (largely unspoken) assumption that regulators were merely enforcing self-evident scientific standards and procedures. These standards and procedures are then applied to non-allopathic modalities whose doctrinal structure is quite different. The FDA, for example, has regulated homeopathy by trying to assimilate it to the allopathic paradigm, which is inappropriate … Attempts to assimilate acupuncture or chiropractic to the allopathic paradigm will be even more misdirected and futile. ... Eventually the public might become so irritated at this regulatory presumption as to demand abolition of medical regulation altogether. While this may seem a purely theoretical possibility, it did indeed happen in the United States 150 years ago. ... This country had no medical licensing for over 50 years, until it was restored in the 1890s."(1) Perhaps it's time, if not to abolish existing licensure, to embrace a rejection of this model for the CAM community.

Paul B. Ginsburg, executive director of the Physician Payment Review Commission, and Ernest Moy, assistant professor of medicine at the University of Maryland School of Medicine conceded in a paper, *Physician Licensure and the Quality of Care*, "Economists have long questioned whether the goal of removing supposedly low-quality practitioners from the market is an appropriate one. Many have advocated replacing licensure with a program that provides consumers with information on practitioners' qualifications and allows them to choose whether to seek services from practitioners not meeting the standards for certification."(2)

According to landmark studies done by Friedman, 1962 and Moore, 1961, "Reviews of licensing suggest that certification and registration arrangements would accomplish the protection of the public as well as the compulsory licensing of practice would." (4)

Harris Coulter suggests "… a further step could be taken, permitting the practice of certain alternative modalities without any licensing requirement at all. This is the situation in England today, where the unlicensed practice of medicine is commonplace and well received by the public, and where the principal curb is the common law prohibition on fraudulent misrepresentation of educational qualifications. In England the patient is assumed to have the good sense to contract for medical services as for other services in life. Are Americans less competent? Why should we not be allowed the same latitude? The English recognize that licensing is usually designed to protect the licensee, not the public. The fact that alternative modalities are more user-friendly than allopathy makes such a course of action even more attractive. Acupuncture, herbalism, homeopathy, and chiropractic are generally recognized as inherently safe. While an alternative practitioner can, of course, be wantonly negligent and thus inflict harm on the patient, the ordinary practice of these disciplines is not dangerous at all. … because allopathy insists on employing the intrinsically toxic medicine, to protect patients, the allopathic licensing requirements should be stricter than those of the alternative modalities." (1)

Georgia addressed this issue in the Official Code of Georgia (OCG) code section 43-1A-2, "It is the purpose of this chapter to ensure that no programs of licensure and certification shall hereafter be imposed upon any profession or business unless required for the safety and well-being of the citizens of the state." However, because a massage association had been denied support for licensure, in part due to their inability to prove harm, in 2003, a sponsor of one of the stymied massage bills introduced HB 628, which took this requirement out of the law. This change, which did not pass (this time), would have paved the way for passage of restrictive licensure without demonstrated need. They also added a statement, "If the business or profession is regulated by more than half of the states, this shall be considered as a factor in determining that the business or profession poses a potential economic, physical, or other type of harm to the health, safety, and welfare of the citizens of the state…" This additional statement effectively makes past paradigm, rather than a need for a law, the determining factor.

There will always be those who fight against your freedom. Those CAM practitioners who pride themselves in federal accreditation, support licensing, and lobby for turf protection, are promoting a risky strategy, imposing burdensome, inefficient, unnecessary overhead on small businesses and entrepreneurs – whose costs are then passed on to consumers. Not only are they interfering with the consumers' constitutional right to make their own healthcare decisions, but as Stanley J. Gross states, "The professional monopolies that result cause the loss of one aspect of economic freedom – namely, the right to choose an occupation." He feels that because of the high value placed on freedom in the United States, the burden of proof should be on the state and license-seekers to show that the loss of freedom is justified by the protection given to the public and "Further, the costs of licensing, which include higher costs of professional services, resistance to innovation in education, training, and services, and maldistribution in the supply and use of professional and para-professional resources, make the price paid by the public for protection even higher and necessitate the requirement for justification."

Young, in his book The Rule of Experts, Occupational Licensing in America, observed "So long as occupational groups continue to regard restrictive licensing laws both as a crucial element of public recognition and as a certain means of acquiring monopoly privileges, more occupations will demand licensure. Without a countervailing pressure, politicians and government administrators will remain only too eager to supply that commodity." (3)

Many, both consumers and professionals, believe that licensing laws are primarily used to protect one group at the expense of other groups. While licensure is presented as a measure to protect the public, it is usually the members of the licensed group who are seeking protection – from actual or potential competitors. It has often been noted that no movement in favor of professional licensing has ever been instigated by the public itself.

Milton Friedman, Nobel Prize Economist said, "The justification for licensure is always the same: to protect the consumer. However...observe who lobbies for imposition or strengthening of licensure. The lobbyists represent the occupation in question, not customers." Ginsburg and Moy contend, "The argument continues that a minimum standard set by government permits the profession to influence the licensing process to erect a restrictive entry barrier and to limit the ways in which its members compete. Thus, consumers pay higher prices for all services." (2)

Stanley Gross, author of <u>Of Foxes and Hen Houses</u> writes, "The history of licensing in the health professions centers on the attempts of special interests to impose or to sabotage a monopoly on the practice of healing. ... The public and most professionals believe that occupational licensing protects service consumers against charlatans and incompetents. ... Rather, the evidence reveals licensing to be a mystifying arrangement that promises protection of the public but that actually institutionalizes a lack of accountability to the public." (4)

Sociologist Marie Haug stated, "Licensing arrangements ... can be characterized less as methods for protecting the public and for providing external social control in the interest of the consumer than as a means for protecting the occupation's market dominance. Indeed, licensing has the unique quality of making a violation of the professional monopoly a punishable crime." (3) The competitors are punished not because they caused injury, didn't know what they were doing, or were not trained. They are punished because they challenged the monopoly. They may deliver better outcomes, be more competent, and be better trained - but trained in a different way than some special interest group has decided they need to be. Therefore they may not be eligible for licensure or unable to pass the licensure exam by regurgitating predetermined answers, even though their clinical skills may be far superior to those licensed.

A former Virginia state official maintained, "The great truth that is never spoken directly, but anybody in the field with two bourbons in them will tell you, is that these boards work primarily to protect the practitioners and have little or nothing to do with protecting the public." (3)

Following a thorough examination of the effects of licensing across a wide range of occupations, David Young concluded, "Occupational regulation has served to limit consumer choice, raise consumer costs, increase practitioner income, limit practitioner mobility, deprive the poor of adequate services, and restrict job opportunities for minorities – all without a demonstrated improvement in quality or safety of the licensed activities." (3)

If registration, certification, or licensure is not the answer, what is?

You are.

Stan Liebowitz, a professor of managerial economics at the University of Texas, in *Why Health Care Costs Too Much*, completed an analysis of the causes of the increase in healthcare costs. He concluded "The major culprit in the seemingly endless rise in health care costs is found to be the removal of the patient as a major participant in the financial and medical choices that are currently being made by others in the name of the patient."

Ronald E. Bachman agreed in his article *Consumer-Driven Health Care: The Future is Now*, published in Benefits Quarterly, Second Quarter 2004. He wrote, "Distorted purchasing decisions and uncontrollable inflation will remain problems in health care so long as someone other than the patient is paying the bill."

Stanley J. Gross, in *Professional Licensure and Quality: The Evidence*, cites Milton Roemer's belief that there are six basic conditions that are necessary for the achievement of high-quality medical care for a population, and includes "fostering an educated public and maintaining a continuing flow of new knowledge." In other words, an informed consumer is necessary to achieve high-quality medical care, not one who is kept ignorant and in the dark, letting others "call the shots."

Michael Novak noted, "In an advanced society, important inequalities of knowledge and technical understanding multiply. Every citizen is incompetent in many areas … It does not follow that rule by experts is an intelligent response to the new inequalities. It is still wise to trust the ordinary wisdom of plain human beings on juries, in the voting booth, in the development of pubic dialogue, and in the ordinary decencies of daily living. So also, it would seem, a wise society trusts individuals to spend their hard-earned dollars as they judge best." (3)

In a nutshell, licensure and regulations do not protect the consumer. Accurate and honest information is a consumer's best protection. The public needs protection from laws that suppress their healthcare choice and restrict information rather than protection from alternative practitioners.

1. *Alternative Medicine: A Challenge to Federal and State Regulators*, Harris L. Coulter, Ph.D., June 10, 1997, paper presented at the Third Annual International Congress of Alternative & Complementary Therapies, Arlington, Virginia.

2. *Physician Licensure and the Quality of Care,* Paul Ginsburg and Ernest Moy, Regulation: The Review of Business and Government. Vol. 15, no. 4, 1992.

3. The Rule of Experts, Occupational Licensing in America. S. David Young, published by the Cato Institute, a public policy research foundation. Washington, D.C. 1987.

4. *The Myth of Professional Licensing,* Stanley J. Gross, American Psychologist. November 1978.

Protecting the Public in Georgia

*"You can only protect **your** liberties in this world by protecting the **other man's freedom.** "*

Clarence Darrow

In spite of research exposing the negative side of licensure and turf protection, several turf-protective CAM bills were introduced and/or passed during recent legislative sessions in Georgia. The lack of research supporting the "protecting the public" concept, the Official Code of Georgia's (OCG) historical suggestions for minimal regulation, and the call for consumer responsibility in healthcare choices, have not always resulted in freedom-friendly legislation.

HB 814, passed in 2000, placed acupuncture under the control of the Medical Board and restricts its practice to persons certified by a single certification agency. Therefore, you have one private organization determining who shall be able to practice acupuncture in Georgia, and the Medical Board, who has historically tried to annihilate acupuncture, as the controlling body.

After numerous attempts and defeats, HB 347 passed in 2003. It restricts CAM therapy, such as acupuncture, homeopathy, nutriceuticals, and mechanical or manual adjustment procedures to be delivered only to animals by Doctors of Veterinary Medicine. Those best trained to treat animals with alternative medicine, i.e. alternative medicine practitioners, will not be able to treat animals, but veterinarians who may have received minimal or no training in alternative medicine may treat them.

In 2003, SB 162 was introduced which would have technically made it possible to charge all CAM practitioners as felons. It did not pass during the 2003-2004 session but I'm sure we will see it again in some form or fashion. A similar bill passed in Florida several years ago and similar bills have been introduced in other states.

On the opposite side of the restrictive and exclusionist registration, certification, and licensure mindset is the consumer-empowering public domain. Should not natural medicine, that which is provided by nature rather than chemical companies, be available to all? Since restrictive and exclusionist registration, certification, and licensure don't really protect the public as claimed, should not another methodology take their place?

As previously discussed, only one CAM bill (HB 749) was introduced in the 1999-2000 session that did not involve turf protection and did not infringe on an individual's right to choose, nor a practitioner's right to practice. A "Cutting Edge" consumer rights and protection bill, the Complementary and Alternative Health Care Freedom of Access Act, was introduced. HB 749 was based on a similar state bill introduced by the Minnesota Natural Health Coalition. The purpose of HB 749 was to "protect the freedom of the individual to choose and receive the healing treatment that the individual desires and deems to correspond with that individual's own view of health and disease, and which the individual deems to be effective in securing that individual's own wellness and to encourage and promote the practice of all healing methods; and to protect the right of health practitioners to practice all forms of health care."

The bill called for certain disclosures, notices, and informed consent of the client before treatment commences. The complementary and alternative healthcare provider was required to provide certain written disclosures and notices, such as the practitioner's title, health care philosophy, and healthcare services available from the practitioner. Disclosure of the practitioner's education, experience and training, and any credentials, continuing education, and professional affiliations related to the complementary and alternative healthcare practiced by the practitioner was also required. A statement that the practitioner is not licensed in the State of Georgia to practice medicine was mandated. Other information was required such as the nature and purpose of the proposed treatment, benefits to be most likely expected from the proposed treatment, and the most common risks associated with the proposed treatment or procedure.

Although the Minnesota Bill passed overwhelmingly, the Georgia bill was stopped in the General Health Subcommittee of the House Health and Ecology Committee and sent to a study committee. The Minnesota coalition made several amendments as it worked its way through the committees, but the intent of the Bill remained unchanged. The full text of the Minnesota Bill and more detailed information about the Minnesota Natural Health Coalition may be found at www.minnesotanaturalhealth.org. You may find Georgia CAM legislation on the Official State of Georgia Web site at www.legis.state.ga.us and www.camaction.org.

As I shared in the intro, CAMA had a public-domain freedom of access bill prepared to introduce in 2001, we honored a request by the Medical Association of Georgia to hold it until the second half of the session with the promise to work together during the summer to develop a joint bill. Well .... after several delays, several meetings, a threat of charging us as felons, a refusal to include several modalities in the legislation, a demand that nothing short of a board would be acceptable, we deduced that a joint bill was not in the stars. We decided to wait until the 2003-4 session to introduce our next freedom of access bill.

Each year brings the introduction of at least one massage licensure bill. Promoted either as a solution for prostitution or as a necessity for public safety, it remains in reality a method of turf protection and guaranteed income for the professional organization. What is not often understood is that most licensure bills by their nature affect other practitioners outside of the targeted profession. The 2004 versions of these bills placed restrictions on CAM therapists other than massage therapists and would have required other bodyworkers such as reflexologists to obtain a massage school education and licensure to practice, even if they had no intention of practicing massage. Hypnotherapists have also been frequently threatened with mental health, psychologist, or other licensure/scope of practice legislation that would infringe on their right to practice, again limiting consumer choices.

The 2003-2004 version of Georgia's freedom of access legislation was termed the *State Planning for Increased Community Access Act* and placed in the House State Planning and Community Affairs Committee to more fully address the total scope of the CAM Access quandary. CAM Freedom of Access is more than a healthcare issue. It is a freedom issue; it is a human rights issue; it is a cultural issue; it is an issue of religious expression; it is an issue of diversity and respect for people's diversity. It is an issue that the state must address in assuring access to a variety of communities.

It is the State's responsibility to lead the way in planning a way to respect the choice, the culture, and the right of self-determination of its citizens. A study done by Georgia State University and reported in the Atlanta Journal-Constitution in February of 1997, showed that out of the total 2,888,774 residents of Cherokee, Clayton, Cobb, DeKalb, Douglas, Fayette, Fulton, Gwinnett, Henry, and Rockdale counties, 267,000 were immigrants. The greatest number resides in DeKalb County (79,100 immigrants). As impressive as these figures are, it is accepted that the immigrant population is grossly under reported. For example, the Vietnamese population is more accurately counted as 50,000 rather than 10,700 and the Nigerian population as 20,000 rather than the reported 3,500. Since the 1970s there has been a 425% increase in foreign-born residents in metro Atlanta. In 1998 alone, 1,814 immigrants resettled in DeKalb County. The Asian community is the fastest-growing group in metro Atlanta and it is estimated that DeKalb will be one of the ten counties in the United States with the largest percentage of Asian-Americans (4.6% of DeKalb's population). In spite of the great influx of immigrants to the state, an organized plan to accommodate their healthcare preferences has not been implemented. HB 1040 is how some legislators chose to meet this challenge.

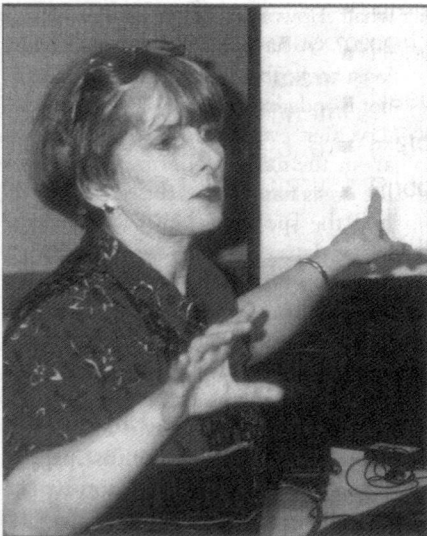

CAM THERAPIES: Complementary and alternative medicine is growing in popularity in the United States, stated Marjorie Robers, MS, RN. Part of the trend can be attributed to America's growing diversity and acceptance of traditional Chinese, African and Native American medicine, while a move toward "natural" foods and remedies is also playing a role. An expert in the field who currently is a consultant at the Atlanta VA Medical Center, Robers said CAM is increasingly eligible for insurance coverage.

Women coming from cultures of modesty will NEVER be comfortable in stirrups when an equally competent lay midwife can assist in their home deliveries. Should they be forced to conform to what allopathic medicine thinks is acceptable because the state has chosen to recognize only the allopathic medical model? Should individuals who come from a culture of home remedies be forced by state law to go without or be forced to utilize chemical drugs? Should politicians and physicians have more control over their bodies than they do? Should a practitioner who wants to share his gift of healing be forced to abandon what he knows and believes and replace it with a modality he is diametrically opposed to? Or should a practitioner with years of education and experience be denied the practice of his/her gift because s/he cannot afford to pay the newly created fees or to jump through the hoops required by the state? If you were a practitioner, how easy would it be for you to pass State Boards after practicing for 40 years? Could you regurgitate the textbook answers called for on the test? After the restrictive acupuncture bill passed, a long-time practitioner of Traditional Chinese Medicine put it this way, "First they steal my culture and then they make it illegal for me to practice my culture."

Because of CAM's recent resurgence in the U.S., because of healthcare's run-away inflation, because over 40 million Americans are uninsured, because of the recognized dangers of allopathic medicine, because of the overuse of antibiotics and other drugs, and because the public is more informed, state protection of CAM access is necessary. Alternative medicine is widely practiced in the State of Georgia without guidelines, without a plan. HB 1040, the *State Planning for Increased Community Access Act*, outlined the state's plan for protecting consumer access and a practitioner's right to work while protecting the consumer through disclosures and disclaimers. It supported a consumer's right to respect their culture and beliefs in choosing their form of healthcare. It supported the CAM Practitioners' right to practice their profession without harassment, while holding them responsible for professional conduct.

In 2004, Georgia legislators had to choose whether they would protect consumers freedom of choice, protect its citizens' right to work, protect the taxpayer from funding unnecessary and costly regulation, and protect Georgia citizens' right to practice their beliefs/culture without state interference. In spite of what we felt was "right,"

HB 1040 did not pass.   Not enough legislators decided that the consumer should have the benefit of all healthcare options. Not enough consumers wanted control over their body. Consumers didn't show up in the numbers needed to voice their concern. Legislators didn't take it upon themselves to speak up for the silent majority.

At the time of this writing, we continue to educate and prepare for re-introduction of health freedom legislation in the 2005-2006 session.

Won't you join us?

Relinquishing Your Responsibilities – Relinquishing Your Rights

"If you need an excuse... any excuse will do."

Marjorie Roberts

Who is responsible for my health? Me, myself, and I.

Sure, a Mac truck over which we have no control may hit us, or we may have inherited genes and familial tendencies we have no control over, but for much of our health status, we have ourselves to thank or blame. During my almost 30 years in nursing I have seen many patients insisting that the doctors, or nurses, or hospital, or whoever, make them well. They discount that the 30 years of cigarette smoking, 20 years of over indulgence in alcohol, or daily consumption of processed and fast food may have invited this encounter with ill health. But then, if it's not the health system's fault for not keeping them well, it must be the fault of the cigarette advertisers for getting them addicted to the nicotine, or the fast pace that doesn't allow them to eat right, or the necessity of having three cars, four televisions, and two computers that makes them work two jobs to "make ends meet" elevating their stress level.

If you need an excuse, any excuse will do.

But there is good news!!!!! People are beginning to sit up and take notice. Organic foods are becoming more and more common and available. We are no longer "kooks" if we do acupressure on Hegu (an acupuncture point between your thumb and index finger) instead of popping aspirin. Smoking has become socially unacceptable. Public health nurses are administering acupuncture to help people quit smoking. Tai Chi has become a household word. Echinacea will soon be found in everyone's medicine cabinet. John Knowles, former president of the Rockefeller Foundation said **"The next major advance in the health of American people will be determined by what the individual is willing to do for themselves."**

We are bombarded daily by television telling us to take medicine for anything that ails us. If we want to eat food that our bodies don't agree with, that's okay, we take magic pills before or drink potions afterward. If we're constipated and don't like to eat fruits and vegetables to keep us regular, that's okay, we'll take laxatives instead. If we have diarrhea, and don't want to blame it on that grease-laden burger, that's okay, we'll take pills instead. If we can't sleep, and don't want to give up the coffee and the blood and guts on the 11 o'clock news, that's okay, we'll just take sleeping pills. When we have a headache from not eating or from running non-stop and don't have time to slow down and take care of ourselves, that's okay, we'll just take aspirin instead.

We certainly must maintain a constant vigilance to keep from being snookered into medicating ourselves toward illness. We have a tendency to not listen to our bodies but instead hush the voices with pills. Benjamin Franklin said "He's the best physician who knows the worthlessness of most medicines." Albert Schweizer said, "We doctors do nothing. We only help and encourage the doctor within." What power we have! We just have to recognize it and act on it. We need to become informed consumers. A man insists on knowing every little thing about a car he's about to buy, but doesn't know about his body or that pill he's popping. A woman can spend a fortune on having special formulas of make-up to put on her face, but organic food is too expensive for her family. A teen places great pride in being up-to-date on the latest pop or rap artist, but doesn't have a clue about attaining a long healthy life.

Our right to choose our healthcare comes with a level of responsibility if we want to do it right and safe and with confidence. We have to make the decision that it is up to us to determine the level of our health. Stop making excuses. Start making changes. Realize that you and your decisions are the key to your health. Become responsible.

Albert Schweizer said, "The greatest discovery of any generation is that human beings can alter their lives by altering the attitudes of their minds." Let's adopt the attitude of accepting responsibility for our health practices. Let's adopt the attitude of setting healthy examples for our children. Let's adopt the attitude that we have the power to alter our lives and health for the better. One of the things we have control over is our attitude. Attitude is our choice.

Get Out Your Plow!

Demand, Insist, Command

"There are two primary **choices** *in life: to accept conditions as they exist, or accept the responsibility for changing them. "*

Denis Waitley

You should now be convinced - there are two healthcare movements movin' on. There is the so-called *Freedom Movement* driven by consumers and the *Restrict Access Movement* driven by special interest groups, predominantly the allopathic medical profession and the pharmaceutical cartel. In Georgia, SB 162, a bill threatening CAM Practitioners with felony charges, was one of the bills that represents the *Restrict Access Movement*. HB 1040 represented the *Freedom Movement*. And when these bills pass or are defeated – it's not over. We must maintain vigilance to maintain that victory.

One of my favorite *movement* quotes is by Frederick Douglas. He said, "If there is no struggle, there is no progress. Those who profess to favor freedom, and yet deprecate agitation, are men who want crops without plowing up the ground. They want rain without thunder and lightning. They want the ocean without the awful roar of its many waters. This struggle may be a moral one; or it may be a physical one; or it may be both moral and physical; but it must be a struggle. Power concedes nothing without a demand. It never did and never will."

Thanks to the Minnesota movement and other freedom fighters that have preceded us, and those who are now working in synchrony, we have a fertile field with which to work. Now it's up to us to plow the ground. Write those letters to your legislators in support of your state's version of freedom of access. If there ever was a time to join your state organization that is working for freedom of access, NOW is the time. Make plans to participate in their events. Donate to their advocacy or lobbyist fund. Become a volunteer.

Let's not let weeds grow. Let's plow and plant and bring down rain to prepare for an abundant crop.

There's been a lot of talk over the past years about freedom of access, how the complementary/alternative medicine practitioners want it; the consumers deserve it; our crumbling health care system needs it. Lots of talk. Lots of *professing* freedom. Not enough doing the work. You know who you are and who you aren't. Those states that have passed freedom bills should be greatly appreciative of a small core group that did the work and paid the price while most sat on the sidelines. Those states who haven't passed freedom legislation must also be greatly indebted to those in other states who have stepped out ahead and set the example.

Those of us who support health freedom of access have heard lots of talk but haven't seen enough movement, enough agitation. Most of the agitation has been the aggravation from the status quo. We want abundant crops - lots of people converted to believing in the benefits of and utilizing CAM. We want the raining down from heaven of acceptance and credibility. We want the ocean swell of support for our right to help consumers with alternative healthcare and to use that healthcare which coincides with their belief system.

But too many haven't wanted the work of plowing that must precede the crops. The thunder and lightning of criticism and scrutiny that accompanies the rain has been too uncomfortable to weather. People do not want to hear the seemingly awful, relentless roar of calls to action over and over again.

We must come to recognize and accept that "power concedes nothing without a demand" and we must demand. We must be ready and willing to plow, to call down thunder and lightning and ROAR - and not stop roaring until we usher in CAM freedom in each of our states.

It is up to us to decide if we want freedom in healthcare choices or just continue to whimper and complain about it and concede to the status quo of having our choices made for us. Perhaps we feel comfortable because we have the knowledge and resources to find an "underground alternative practitioner" who can provide care for our family. Perhaps we don't even know that our choices are limited. Benjamin Rush, M.D., signer of the Declaration of Independence and physician to George Washington predicted, "unless we put medical freedom into the Constitution, the time will come when medicine will organize into an undercover dictatorship... To restrict the art of healing to one class of men and deny equal privileges to others will constitute the Bastille of medical science. All such laws are un-American and despotic and have no place in a republic... The Constitution of this republic should make special privilege for medical freedom as well as religious freedom." (1)

In Georgia, the 1997 passage of SB 341, sponsored by Senator Gochenour, was a beginning in shifting the regulatory focus from protecting medical orthodoxy to protecting the consumer's interest. However, the bill did not go far enough. It stated that, "the individual shall have the right to be treated for any illness or disease which is potentially life threatening or chronically disabling ...with any experimental or nonconventional medical treatment that such individual desires or the legal representative of such individual authorizes..." but limits the providers to only those persons licensed to practice medicine, thereby eliminating treatment by homeopaths, chiropractors, acupuncturists, naturopaths, and other healthcare providers. This takes it out of the realm of patient choice. It blocks the individual's unrecognized legal right, "the right to maximize the individual's opportunity for healing disease." (2)

Healthcare choices in most states are limited in a number of ways. In a few states, physicians who are licensed to practice medicine can now provide unconventional therapies requested by patients under certain circumstances. Most other practitioners who suggest, recommend, or prescribe any type of therapy may be charged with the practice of medicine. Michael Cohen in the Arizona Law Review states, "... when courts find that alternative and complementary providers have exceeded their legislative authorization or scope of practice and have unlawfully practiced "medicine," the decisions rarely reflect a clear vision of legislative wisdom or public policy. Rather, the decisions reflect confusion over scope of practice boundaries, deference to medical dominance and orthodoxy, and references to unorthodox providers as "cultist," "fringe," "marginal," and "quacks."(2) He goes on to say "...the current regulatory scheme embodies a strong dose of paternalism in aiming to protect patients from their own ill-advised choices....licensing statutes grant medical doctors unlimited authority, and nonmedical competitors a more limited authority to help patients heal." "Such strong paternalism is unjustified, given that consumers can and do choose to address their health needs, in many states, by visiting licensed chiropractors, acupuncturists, naturopaths, and others, and by relying on self-care and nutrition, including dietary supplements which they purchase in health food stores."(2)

Cost is still another factor in limiting your choice in healthcare provider. Due to numerous rules and regulations, third-party reimbursement is only allowable for "privileged" occupations. Protection of the public is often cited as the reason for these regulations. However, Deborah Haas-Wilson, associate professor of economics at Smith College, relates, "the major justification for regulating health professionals is to increase the quality of their services and thus to protect the interests of uninformed healthcare consumers" but "... the regulations developed by self-regulating health professionals increasingly are being perceived as a means to serve their self-interests, rather than the 'public interest'." She states, "...studies show that a self-regulating profession may set minimum quality standards excessively high or may increase its members' incomes at the cost of reducing consumer welfare" and "In general, the empirical research suggests consensus on the need to deregulate the market for health care professionals' services."(3) Perhaps a statement in *The Pharos of Alpha Omega Alpha Honor Medical Society* journal sums it up; "Furthermore, the tremendous sums of money paid to alternative practitioners could then go directly to physicians and the mainstream health care economy."(4)

"Worldwide, seventy to ninety percent of health care uses self-care or care based on an alternative tradition or practice; only ten to thirty percent is based on biomedicine (drugs). Alternative and complementary therapies prevail because chronic, debilitating conditions such as arthritis, allergies, pain, hypertension, cancer, depression, cardiovascular, and digestive problems account for seventy percent of the healthcare budget, and affect 33 million Americans, 9 million of whom cannot work, attend school, or maintain a household." (3) Many health care providers also recognize the deficiencies in our present healthcare system which is predominated by pharmaceuticals and surgery. Dr. Leaf writes in the <u>Journal of the American Medical Association</u>, "I think there is much to indicate that a healthcare system, the goal of which is to prevent illness and to promote health, will cost less than the present system that basically operates to respond to the presence of illness, often with very costly diagnostic and therapeutic interventions... Most compelling to me is that the nearly total preoccupation of physicians today with these palliative interventions will do nothing for the next generation of 30-, 40-, or 50-year-olds, ..." (5) A study from the Center for Pharmaceutical Economics, College of Pharmacy, The University of Arizona in Tucson reported, "Drug-related morbidity and mortality was estimated to cost $76.6 billion in the ambulatory setting in the United States." and "The cost of drug-related morbidity and mortality.... should be considered in health policy decisions with regard to pharmaceutical benefits."(6) Is it any wonder that the American public is looking to alternative medical care for some answers?

What still perplexes me is why the American public isn't paying more attention and DEMANDING answers and accountability.

Now we must ask ourselves as both practitioners and consumers -

Are we comfortable with CAM being controlled by those whose philosophy and approach to health/disease is diametrically opposed to that of most CAM therapies?

Are we comfortable following in the path of allopathic medicine, pursuing the formation of an unnecessary licensing board in order to fit in with "mainstream?"

As consumers, do we want to be restricted in our choice of practitioner, forced to choose among those approved by the Medical Board… or any other state regulatory board?

As consumers, do we lack the intelligence and willingness to make our own decision?

As practitioners, do we want to practice to the full extent of our training and capabilities or do we want to be restricted by those who don't have a clue about the philosophy of natural medicine?

During one of our joint MAG/CAMA meetings at the MAG office, I noticed that their lobbyist had printed out much of the CAMA Web site and was well versed on its content. How many of you who profess to be advocates of CAM have visited the CAMA Web site or your state organization's Web site, much less read/studied their mission or the legislative information?

Do you know who your legislators are; have you contacted them, worked on a campaign, or sent a campaign contribution? Check your Secretary of State's Web site, www.followthemoney.org, or www.vote-smart.org, where campaign contributions are listed. You'll find lots of medical organization and pharmaceutical company contributions - especially to members of the health committees. Its not buying votes, it's supporting those who share your mission and philosophy. The opponents of freedom of access have understood the necessity of supporting the legislators who support their monopolistic mission. Many freedom advocates have not yet reached the realization that you must support those policy-makers who are sensitive to the preservation of your rights to choose alternative medicine.

CAMA and other state Freedom organizations have many dedicated members and volunteers that support their work, both through their membership and volunteer work - because they understand they are really supporting their work - their existence, their freedom to choose, and a wealth of education/information. To these champions (both practitioners and consumers), other practitioners and consumers owe their existence. Now, the freedom seekers who have been sitting on the sidelines need to step up to the plate.

It's difficult to testify on behalf of the millions of consumers who use CAM throughout the US when only thousands are involved in any movements. We won't get results when we substitute excuses for action. And when you need an excuse – any excuse will do.

I can't afford it: Most freedom groups charge about $2-3/month for basic supporters, hardly enough to break the piggy bank and much less than your monthly cable bill.

I don't get any clients from my affiliation with the Group: I have yet to find in any mission statement that the Group is existing to market your business for you. Most freedom groups are working to keep all CAM Practitioners in practice.

I live too far away/too busy to attend the lectures/events/Capitol: So what? Your inability to physically participate is all the more reason for you to support in a manner that you can – prayer, money, and membership.

I keep forgetting to join/renew: That works for the first 2 years or the first 20 invitations, whichever comes first. If it's really the case, you definitely need to protect CAM because it's your only hope for restoring your mind.

If we don't get to work, we will not be in a position to gain or maintain Freedom legislation in our country, but will be forced to compromise for laws that are not in the best interest of the consumer and/or CAM Practitioner. Or worse yet, we will have no choice as the medical and pharmaceutical cartels introduce their own bill with NO input from the CAM Community.

Choose to take responsibility for your future or continue to work away - too busy, too uninformed, too apathetic, too righteous, too victimized to get involved. Call your state organization and find out what you can do or sit on your derrière and let s_it happen. Your response or lack thereof will determine the direction of healthcare freedom.

As Frederick Douglas said, "If there is no struggle, there is no progress. Those who profess to favor freedom, and yet deprecate agitation, are men who want crops without plowing up the ground. They want rain without thunder and lightning. They want the ocean without the awful roar of its many waters. This struggle may be a moral one; or it may be a physical one; or it may be both moral and physical; but it must be a struggle. Power concedes nothing without a demand. It never did and never will."

Get out your plow and get to work. Learn to not be afraid of the thunder and lightening. Heed the beckoning roar or the call to action! You can join in the struggle with a demand for freedom in health care choices or sit back on the stool of "do nothing" and kiss your health care freedom goodbye.

(1) *Alternative Medicine: The Definitive Guide*, compiled by The Burton Goldberg Group, Future Medicine Publishing.

(2) Cohen, Michael H., *Arizona Law Review*, The University of Arizona College of Law, Vol. 38, No. 1, Spring 1996.

(3) Haas-Wilson, Deborah, The Regulation of Health Care Professionals Other Than Physicians, *Cato Institute Regulation Publication*.

(4) Erickson, Joel Keith, <u>The Language of Acupuncture: Should Western Physicians Learn It?</u> *The Pharos of Alpha Omega Alpha Honor Medical Society,* Fall '95.

(5) Leaf, A., MD, <u>Preventive Medicine for Our Ailing Health Care System</u>, *JAMA*, 2/3/93.

(6) Johnson, J.A., MSc., Bootman, J. L., PhD., <u>Drug-Related Morbidity and Mortality</u>, *Arch Intern Med*, 10/9/95.

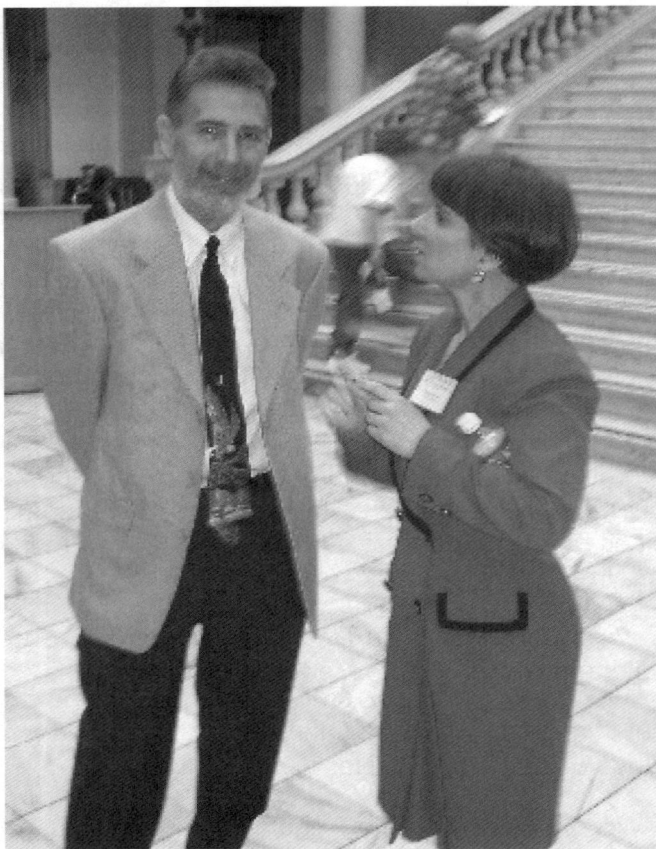

Myself visiting with a guest at the Georgia State Capitol during one of our education days.

A Majority Makes It So...NOT.

*"There's not power in numbers;
there's power in organized numbers."*

Marjorie Roberts

Gang mentality. Majority rules. The masses. The golden rule (those with the gold – rule). A majority of money, a majority of people, a majority of power.

When are facts really facts and when are they facts because the majority or group in power decides they are? On occasion, facts change because of new legitimate scientific discoveries. More often, facts change because a majority decides to make it so. We take a vote to decide what is correct, truth, fact. And we vote with our money, our power, and our influence.

I see it in the media. Advertisements disguised as news stories to manipulate public opinion. Movie stars promoting products in so-called interviews without divulging their financial interests in the products. Pharmaceutical drugs being falsely advertised through TV commercials, but by the time the FDA calls them on it, the commercial run is over and they go on to the next deceptive commercial. Pharmaceutical companies design commercials which condition consumers to demand that their doctors give them the latest drug for whatever real or imaginary problem the commercial convinces them they have. And of course the drug is "proven" to be effective. After all, the studies show that the "majority" of sufferers suffer no more. The drug cartel is hoping that enough of the public is too ignorant, too busy, too apathetic, or too preoccupied with life to recognize the lies and deception. Those who have purchased the media may decide what the "facts" should be and then proceed to manipulate you into agreeing with their summation.

I see it in the religious community. I used to go to church very faithfully, usually twice on Sunday, almost every Wednesday night, and sometimes even for the Tuesday morning special service. (In retrospect, a definite out-of-balance life.) I expected truth from the preacher – don't laugh; remember I said I was out of balance. The (white) preacher man had convinced vulnerable women to join his sex orgies under the guise of "ascending to a new spiritual level." No, not me. When real truth started to reveal itself and people began leaving the church, he tried to convince the congregation that whites were leaving because the church was becoming too "black." Those who left were mostly white members because whites were the ones in the inner circle who first discovered the lie, as well as being the victims. He announced this "fact" one morning from the pulpit in the presence of all, including children. And of course he had an entourage of about 12 other pastors confirming the statement by their silence.

That was my cue to make an appointment with my individual pastor. I knew several white members who by that time had left the church and I knew the reason why. It had nothing to do with black or white but had to do with lies and deception. And my analysis was that even if whites were leaving the church because of "black" infiltration (which they were not), to speak that in the presence of vulnerable, impressionable children with delicate self-esteems showed total lack of caring for the very group of people he supposedly was there to elevate. But alas, my personal (black) preacher didn't even have the balls to stand up for his "own people." He made some lame excuse that things were being taken care of. I went to one more service but it made me so nauseous that I never went back again.

I still have friends that go to that church and the pervert is still preaching from the pulpit. They still believe that he is truth because he has enough others around him saying that it is so. They lack the where-with-all to think on their own; it's much easier that way. Much more comfortable. And don't tell me this is an isolated incidence; just look to Tammy Faye and Jim Baker, Jim Jones, the Catholic Church, and Jimmy Swaggert, then tell me that deception is not rampant in the church. Their ministries are built on lies and deception.

I see it in the legal system. In 1973, the Georgia Attorney General determined that a physician performing acupuncture could be prosecuted for "unprofessional conduct." Acupuncture was considered unscientific, voodoo, placebo, and certainly NOT the practice of medicine. Then, in 1991, the AG determined that only a physician could practice acupuncture in Georgia. Acupuncture didn't change; it helped people 5,000 years ago, just as it did in 1973 and 1991, and does today and will tomorrow. The facts changed because those in power decided to change them. The allopathic medical monopoly discounted alternative medicine and has historically tried to annihilate it, acupuncture among them. In the famous Eisenberg study of 1990, the medical establishment discovered that $17.3 billion was being spent on alternative medicine practitioners. Then all of a sudden it had some legitimacy; the medical establishment began to "integrate" it into their practices, and of course the plan was put into place for allopathy to control it.

I see it in the political arena. Where the majority of money often makes it so. Wheelin' and dealin' is the name of the game. As of this writing, Georgia is the only state in the union that does not have prescriptive privileges for Nurse Practitioners. Are 49 other states and the District of Columbia wrong? Do they not know the facts? Why does the Georgia Medical Association oppose this legislation every time it comes up for a vote? Could it be money? or control? Do they think that the Nurse Practitioners in Georgia are so inferior that they should not have the same practice privileges as they do in all the other states? And how many legislators have really studied the issue – or does the legislation ever get to the chamber for a vote?

Decisions are being made, not on facts but on perceptions or coercion through money, power, or numbers. The reality of this kind of thinking, this mentality, revealed itself to me in a most deliberate and personal manner. This experience prompted me to look at this whole arena of how truths are determined and changed.

A friend and colleague, in preparation for a presentation she was about to deliver, showed her PowerPoint slides to me on the way to make copies for handouts. Glancing at them, I noticed a grammatical error which I pointed out to her. She had used "whose moving my cheese" rather than "who's moving my cheese." As she appeared somewhat unclear about my correction, I explained that "who's" is the contraction of "who is" and was the proper spelling for this particular statement. She thanked me and went on her way, presumably to correct the mistake. A few hours later, she informed me that she had consulted the Internet and a fellow colleague and most assuredly, I was in error. The Internet said that *whose* was possessive and therefore they decided by majority, that *whose* was the correct form. After all, she was talking about who the cheese belonged to, who possessed it. Pointing out the fact that the word was not used possessively in this sentence did not dissuade her. It was voted on; majority ruled; the presentation and handouts were delivered with the improper grammar.

The fact that both she and her colleague hold Master's Degrees (one in education), may have given them the extra confidence and false perception of themselves as experts in an area they obviously are not. One of the participants IS expert in various aspects of clinical nursing, but not grammar. If I were in need of a competent clinical nurse there would be few better than her. She is top notch, stays current in her practice, is compassionate, and truly cares for her patients. The other is an administrator and although I don't relate to her authoritarian style and we've had more than one sparring event, she is a get-it-done manager and has a passion and dedication to nursing that must be respected and I count myself as one of her admirers.

Some facts I believe are absolute and some are not. Although our sky may not always be azure blue, it won't be green. Although one might challenge the power of numbers, two plus two will always equal four. Although the meaning of our words may change among groups of people and "bad" may actually mean "good," whose will remain possessive and who's will mean who is.

When facts are nothing but someone's perception or misperception— they can be changed. They don't change on their own; they are changed by informed people, by trailblazers, by thinkers outside-the-box.

It may be a little disconcerting to some, knowing that some facts can be changed by majority rule. But it is also an opportunity.

In one of my "voice your choice" arguments with one of the legislators, we were discussing the control that the medical monopoly had over consumer choice. The legislator, who is black, insisted that the Medical Association has the power and little 'ole me was not going to change things. My response, "Aren't you glad your civil rights leaders didn't feel the same way – or you'd still be sitting in the back of the bus."

The civil rights movement challenged people's beliefs. That blacks did not deserve equal access, equal rights, and equal treatment under the law was a misperception perpetuated by those who stood to gain financially and socially. Because the majority (or those in power) felt blacks were inferior did not make it so, but yet it <u>was</u> so. A majority made it so. Only the faithfulness and perseverance of black leaders of that day helped usher in the genuine truth. The movement was an opportunity to correct the "facts." And that opportunity continues today.

And so it is with healthcare. We have the opportunity to set the record straight. The majority is shifting the truth. No longer is alternative medicine the second-class citizen it once was, used only by so-called weirdoes. It is on its way to becoming an equal member of the healthcare family. Consumers are discovering that both alternative medicine and allopathy have their advantages and disadvantages and that both are valuable. The truth of alternative medicine as invalid can shift because indeed it was not truth to begin with, only a misrepresentation, made fact by power and money. The new truth is now being exposed, again by power, but by the power of the masses rather than the power of the select few through money and influence.

Evaluate your truths – they aren't all true. Evaluate what appears to be untruths – some of them are truths misrepresented for someone else's gain. King Solomon said, "a man who judges a matter before he hears it is a fool." Judge a matter after hearing the arguments for yourself – don't automatically take another's interpretation. The majority is not always right and the lone voice crying in the wilderness is not always the crazy one. Choose your truth based on facts, evaluation, and discernment.

One of the most critical areas that you must discern truth is in the area of your healthcare. Your body, your health, and your choice of healthcare are your responsibility. Make those choices based on factual truths, not on truths orchestrated by money, the pharmaceutical cartel, politics, and media clips.

Notes

Your Washington DC Congressman or Congresswoman:

_____

His/Her contact information:

Your two United States Senators:

_____ and _____

Their contact information:

Your State Senator: _____

His/Her contact information:

Your State Representative/Assemblyperson:

_____

His/Her contact information:

Frequently Asked Questions About
Freedom of Access Legislation

A special **thank you** to the Florida Health Freedom Action organization that provided much of the material for this chapter, the National Health Freedom Action for their continual encouragement, and to the other state organizations who so freely contributed their perspectives.

Although there will be slight variations from state to state, the following talking points will assist in your understanding of the issue. It will facilitate your communication with legislators and others regarding the need for this legislation and the concepts on which it is based. Share this information with each and every lover of freedom that you meet.

~~~~~~~~~~~~~~~~

What are complementary and alternative therapies?

Complementary and alternative therapies, also referred to as CAM (Complementary/Alternative Medicine), include therapies outside the realm of allopathic (drugs/surgery/radiation) medicine. These therapies include but are not limited to homeopathy, herbal therapies, exercise/movement, vitamins, relaxation methods, lifestyle, diet, imagery, energy healing, biofeedback, and folk remedies (remember your mother's chicken soup for a cold?). CAM emphasizes preventive and natural practices. Natural practices include healing modalities that work with and enhance the body's inherent ability to heal. Healthcare activities that involve a real danger of significant harm are regulated and licensed by the state, and for that reason are prohibited under this legislation.

CAM may be used with allopathic medical care or used as an alternative to allopathic medicine, such as massage instead of a sleeping pill, hypnotherapy instead of a nicotine patch, or homeopathy instead of anti-histamines.

CAM practitioners are currently practicing in many states. Why is this law needed?

Under the current law, most CAM practitioners can be found to be in technical violation of the law because state licensing boards might consider their activities to be the "practice of medicine" or the practice of another licensed profession. Most states, with the exception of Minnesota, Rhode Island, and California, do not recognize unlicensed healthcare professions and may use the full force of the state's police power to suppress these healthcare practices. In fact, CAM practitioners can be prosecuted even if their practices have nothing to do with medicine in the conventional sense and they have caused no physical or mental harm.

This policing action has had a chilling effect on the growth of healthcare choice in the United States - at a time when more people than ever are seeking preventive and natural, non-toxic, non-invasive healthcare. These state policies curtail consumer freedoms by putting all natural practitioners, as well as those doctors and institutions that would hire them, at risk of closure and prosecution.

There are thousands of natural healthcare providers practicing throughout the United States with thousands of clients. The studies of use of alternative healthcare by the National Institutes for Health and Harvard infer that millions of otherwise law-abiding citizens may be being pushed outside of the law by outdated public policy when they choose an unlicensed practitioner.

Because of this legal threat of prosecution, CAM practitioners have been inhibited and the public has been deprived of important information. CAM practitioners are reluctant to hold themselves out to the public, to develop practitioner standards, and to disclose their credentials to clients. Thus, the public is denied access to information that would allow them to make informed choices about CAM practitioners and the theories on which their modalities are based. Existing laws discourage many individuals from training to become CAM practitioners and slows the development of CAM practices. These same laws discourage clients of CAM practitioners, who are also patients of licensed healthcare providers, from having their licensed providers and their CAM practitioners communicate with each other. This inhibits integrated care for consumers. Almost 80%

of CAM clients do not tell their licensed provider that they are consulting CAM practitioners.

Medical licensing laws in the United States were developed because conventional medical care utilizes high-risk therapies such as surgery, radiation, and pharmacology.

For example, in Georgia, OCG 43-34-26, the definition of medicine states:

"If any person shall hold himself out to the public as being engaged in the diagnosis or treatment of disease or injuries of human beings, or shall <u>suggest</u>, <u>recommend</u>, or <u>prescribe</u> <u>any</u> form of treatment for the palliation, relief, or cure of <u>any</u> physical or mental ailment of any person, with the intention of receiving therefor, either directly or indirectly, any fee, gift, or compensation whatsoever … shall be deemed to be practicing medicine ..." (emphasis mine)

Most states have similar broad scope of practice laws for the practice of medicine. It is this broad language that is the problem. Under this definition, recommending an herb is viewed as the practice of medicine. To put it another way, our current laws do not distinguish between brain surgery and non-invasive practices that hold no demonstrable risk of harm.

If a CAM practitioner has formal training and is certified in his/ her healing art, doesn't that mean s/he can practice legally?

CAM practitioners who have formal training and are certified have met certain requirements that demonstrate proficiency in their healing modality. However, certification exams are administered by healing art organizations themselves and not by the state. For example, the National Guild of Hypnotists certifies hypnotherapists. Whether or not the State licenses a profession is a completely separate issue … and a business license is yet another issue.

Having a "license" means that a practitioner is approved by the state to legally practice within the scope of his/her license. Some CAM practitioners such as chiropractors are licensed by the state. However, many CAM practitioners are not licensed, even though they may be well trained, experienced, and certified in their modality. Under Freedom Legislation, CAM practitioners who are not licensed by the state will be allowed to practice their healing arts as long as they do not perform activities that create a real danger of significant harm to their clients. Of equal importance, for the first time they will be required to give information to their clients about their training and experience, including certification in their modality.

How will the CAM Freedom of Access Act benefit consumers?

The Act frees CAM practitioners to practice openly, while specifying that they cannot perform certain medical activities or put their clients at a true risk of significant harm. For example, CAM practitioners will not be allowed to perform surgery, prescribe certain drugs, recommend that clients discontinue drugs that were prescribed by a licensed provider, or use or prescribe radiation. For the benefit of consumers, the Act requires CAM practitioners to disclose to clients their training and experience, to explain the rationale behind their method of treatment, to make absolutely clear to their clients that they are not "licensed" by the state, and to keep records showing that they have disclosed this information to their clients.

The Act creates an atmosphere that will improve public safety. (1) the Act explicitly prohibits CAM practitioners from treating clients in a way that causes or creates a genuine risk of significant harm and it explicitly forbids certain medical activities; (2) it requires CAM practitioners to disclose their training and experience and the rationale behind their treatment; (3) by allowing CAM practitioners to practice openly, the Act facilitates the development and growth of organizational societies for practitioners of those therapies, which will improve the training and monitoring of their practitioner members; (4) by bringing CAM practitioners out of the shadows and giving their clients written information about themselves and their CAM therapy, the Act encourages and facilitates consumer communication between their licensed healthcare professionals and their CAM practitioners.

Since some licensed healthcare providers can use CAM in conjunction with their standard treatments, why isn't that enough?

Licensed providers are not always trained in CAM modalities, most are not intimately familiar with the range of modalities and some do not recognize or approve of CAM modalities. Individuals trained in CAM modalities are an important source of healthcare to members of the public. Sixty-nine percent of Americans use CAM modalities, most often for minor ailments or serious conditions for which conventional medicine can offer little in the way of therapeutic help. These problems include chronic pain, anxiety, chronic fatigue syndrome, sprains and muscle strains, addictive problems, arthritis, and headaches. Over 95% of consumers who now use CAM modalities do so in conjunction with and not as a replacement for licensed healthcare.

While many physicians recognize and approve of CAM modalities, 60% of surveyed physicians referred their patients to CAM practitioners rather than performing those therapies themselves. Only 23% actually performed CAM modalities themselves.

What if a consumer has a problem with a CAM practitioner?

First, the consumer should talk to their practitioner and try to work out any problem with him or her. If that proves unsatisfactory, they can contact the practitioner's certifying/professional organization. As a last resort, the Act does nothing to stop a consumer from seeking civil relief against a CAM practitioner or, depending on the nature of the problem, asking for action by the Department of Health, Solicitor General, Composite Board of Medical Examiners, or other State Professional Board.

As always, responsibility ultimately rests with the consumer, for wisely choosing a practitioner who has good training, experience, and skills. The disclosure and disclaimer mandates of this Act facilitate this process.

What can happen if a CAM practitioner practices in a prohibited area, creates a real risk of significant harm to a client, or doesn't give a client the written information required?

Any CAM practitioner who practices in a prohibited area (such as performing surgery or discontinuing prescribed medications) or who creates a real risk of significant harm, is denied the protections of the Act and may be treated in the same way they could have been before the Act was passed. The offending practitioner may be criminally prosecuted, subjected to civil fines, be ordered by a court to stop the forbidden practices, and obliged to reimburse the State for the costs of legal proceedings against him/her.

Any CAM practitioner who fails to provide written information about himself/herself or his/her therapy methodology, or fails to inform clients that he/she is not "licensed" by the state, may be fined civilly, ordered by a court to fulfill these requirements, and obliged to reimburse the State for the costs of legal proceedings needed to force compliance with the law.

America Used to be Synonymous with Freedom

Now America is the Name of my Dog

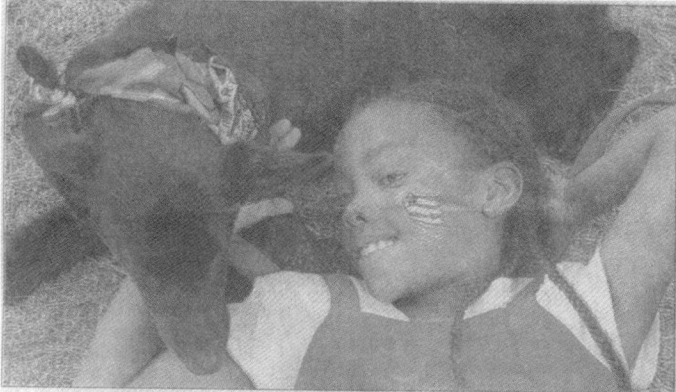

Aliya Parker, **7**, of **Decatur**, is accompanied by her new dog, which she named America, and her family at the benefit for New York firefighters on the city's square.

America is still referred to as the land of the free and home of the brave. It's the principle our country was founded on.

A few years back, I received a call from Mara. She was a native of Italy, had married an American GI, and had recently moved to the United States with him. She called CAMA in search of alternative practitioners. She couldn't find them listed in the phone book or the yellow pages. In her home country of Italy they practice in the open, listed in the phone book. When I shared with her the situation in Georgia, the fact that alternative practitioners practice under a cloud of potential felony charges and so often don't advertise but choose to practice quietly, she was in awe. Her comment: "But I thought America was a free country."

I feel more than blessed to live in America. I believe many foreigners feel the same as they risk life and limb to migrate legally and/or illegally to our shores. I attended school in Mexico during my nursing education and participated in medical missions to Honduras and the

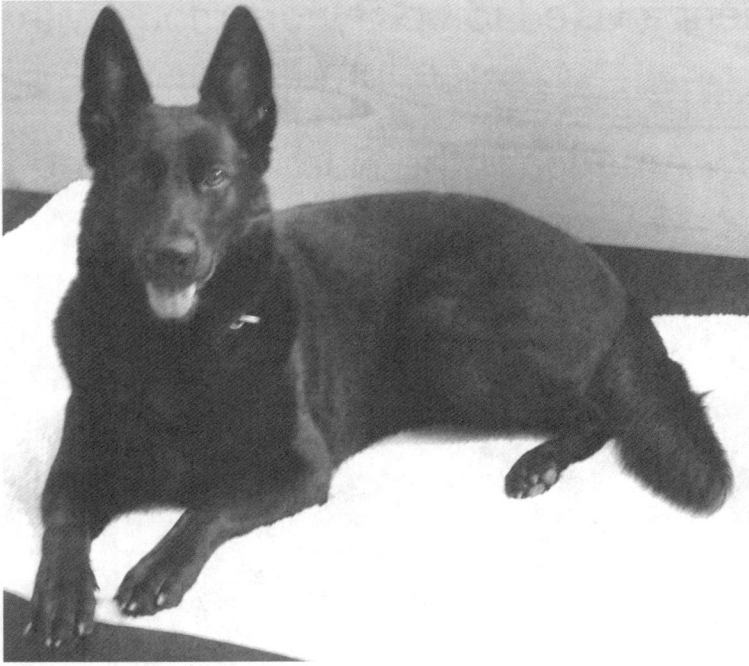

Dominican Republic through my church. I received some of my acupuncture training in Sri Lanke. It was quite an eye-opener to see the lack of basic necessities for the masses. No electricity after 5 PM, no hot water except on Tuesdays and Thursdays, and sometimes no water at all. During one of my missions, I had the good fortune of having the only cat in the place sleeping on the bottom of my bed to keep the mice and rats away. Armed militia on the street corners confirmed my good luck of being born in America. It is experiences such as these that make me determined to do what I can to protect the American way of life.

But sometimes we forget that the American way of life is not only two cars in every garage and a TV in every room. The American way of life is freedom – freedom to choose where you live, where you work, whom you marry, if you marry, who provides your healthcare, whether you accept healthcare, even the freedom to choose to make your own choices or let someone else make choices for you. And that freedom, which our forefathers fought for, helped assure the standard of living we enjoy today. Without freedom, people are oppressed. Oppression stifles productivity. Lack of productivity leads to poverty and disenchantment.

Some say that one must give up individual freedom to gain security. I say that individual freedom must be maintained to experience true security. I am not willing to buy the line that I must choose between freedom and so-called-security. There comes a time when the bennies promised in the name of security do not compensate for the loss of freedom. In the field of healthcare for example, we are often encouraged to give up our rights to choose our healthcare provider in exchange for the security of having "affordable" insurance coverage. How many horror stories have you heard about the erosion of this security when upon illness it's discovered that the coverage doesn't exist, is less than expected, or requires an astronomical co-pay. Or is it fair to require that you give up your right to enlist a naturopath as your healthcare provider? Instead, it is demanded that you use allopathic medicine because it has been determined that you can only be "secure" in their "proven" method of treatment? And of course after years of allopathic therapy, you find the answer to your malady with a naturopath. And yet, if we concede that the choices made for us are true and correct, is there still not something that rubs against the grain of freedom and liberty, when you have no choice in those choices?

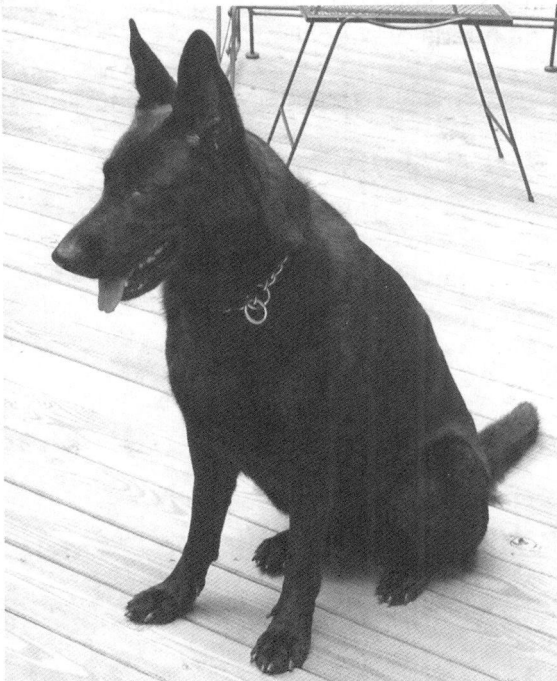

My Miss America, who I received as a blessing when she was 2 years old.

Someone sent me a joke about two dogs. Maybe one's name was America, I don't remember. America was heading to Mexico and the Mexican dog, Pedro, was heading to the United States. They met at the Rio Grande. America asked Pedro why he was headed for the United States. The dog shared how he so looked forward to having hot running water, electricity 24 hours a day, and a clean dry bed to sleep in. It was understandable as to why someone would want to come to the United States. But the Mexican dog could not understand why someone from America would want to go to Mexico. America said it was simply this, "I just want to be able to bark". He was feeling the impact of freedom-stealing actions in America.

He was willing to exchange some of his security for freedom, in this case freedom of speech. America wanted freedom of speech; Mara, from Italy, wanted freedom to choose her healthcare. What freedoms are you willing to give up for a false sense of security?

So here I'll go again with another comment on licensure and those who diligently seek it. Is the promise of the security offered with licensure, such as insurance re-imbursement worth the loss of autonomy? Is monopoly protection a fair exchange for being controlled by a group of people, put in a box, stifled innovation, and the freedom to adapt your therapy to the needs of your client?

Without due diligence our freedoms will continually be siphoned away.

So what are YOU going to do about it?

Freedom - The Word of the Hour

Self-determination, choice, liberty, free will. Freedom by any other name is still a treasure. A treasure that we often don't treasure. A treasure that is often challenged or lost in the quest for security.

That quest for security has never been so evident as it has been since the September 11 tragedy and its resulting avalanche of events challenged our safety and security.

We proclaim freedom as one of the virtues that separates us from many other countries. But we must be forever diligent, lest our freedoms be stolen while we practice apathy or remain uninformed. And we must be forever on guard, lest we be too willing in the name of security to give our freedom away.

We are quick to act when someone from the "outside" attempts to steal our freedom but often don't act at all when the thievery is from "within." Sometimes the thievery is so subtle that we don't even notice; it comes with no publicity. Sometimes we're not told the truth, but a distorted version; our freedom is stolen in the name of "protecting the public." We are convinced that giving up our freedom is a fair exchange for the assurance of protection, security, letting someone else be responsible. Such is the case with healthcare freedom.

In this land of the free, we don't have the freedom to decide who we receive our healthcare from – even if we pay for it. As a healthcare practitioner, we don't have the freedom to enter into a private contract to provide healthcare to another consenting adult. It's hard to imagine that some really accept that others should have more say over our bodies than we do ourselves. We have the right to choose an abortion claiming we can do with our body as we please, but we don't have the right to choose natural healthcare from a naturopath or homeopath. We're given credit to have the intelligence to sit on a jury, consider the facts as presented and determine if someone else lives or dies but can't decide how we want to live. Does this make sense?

Our access is restricted through laws advanced by special interest groups. Florida has made the practice of all unlicensed healthcare providers (homeopaths, herbalists, etc.) a felony. North Carolina introduced a similar unlicensed healthcare provider bill that did not pass. We defeated a Georgia bill that would have made the unlicensed practice of 16 additional health professions a felony (the practice of medicine is already a felony). It passed the Senate but we were able to stop it in the House. Often the rational for restricting our choice is the old rallying call of "protecting the public." We must be protected from the possibility of making poor choices. I believe that the restriction of our healthcare choice has more to do with protecting turf than protecting the public. It all comes down to control and money.

After we knew smoking was hazardous to our health – did we make it illegal? No, we did put a warning on the package and left it up to the individual – free choice. A decision also probably based on control and money; the control of the tobacco companies on public policy through the use of money. What happened when we tried to make alcohol consumption illegal during prohibition? When a law is oppressive, especially when it doesn't make sense, people will disrespect and disobey that law. What happened when Rosa Parks decided that the law commanding her to sit on the back of the bus or give up her seat to a white man was unfair? What is happening even though alternative practitioners are technically in violation of the law? Both alternative practitioners and the people that utilize them break the law. Because the law does not make sense, is oppressive, and is blatantly unfair.

If we want to gain our freedom of access in Georgia and other states as they did in MN, RI and CA, we must become informed and retire our apathy. We must ACT.

As President of CAMA, I received an anonymous, unsolicited e-mail. "I don't attend events or belong to CAMA, but I vote. And if I want to try some new Emotional Freedom Technique or Allergy Elimination Treatment, I damn well better have that right. Is this a free country, or isn't it? That's what I have to say to the state legislature – a Georgia voter."

Although I applaud her (assume female) for taking the time to express her opinion and her commitment to vote, this in itself will do little to assure the freedom she so strongly desires. I would first ask her if she knows how her legislators voted on prior freedom of access issues. Is she an informed voter or does she simply think she did her job because she voted? Did she communicate her opinion to her legislators or just to me? And did she follow up to see if they voted like she wanted them to or said they would? She makes a point to mention that she doesn't belong to CAMA or attend their events. If she does support freedom of access to CAM in Georgia, I find it interesting that she declares her non-support of the one organization in Georgia that is working on behalf of her beliefs. I would tell her that there's not power in numbers; there's power in <u>organized</u> numbers.

The CAM community, both consumers and practitioners, must understand that they have a responsibility for the future or demise of CAM access. Invite your friends, family and neighbors to become involved in their state freedom organization. If you are a CAM practitioner, invite your clients to become involved. If you are a CAM consumer, invite your healthcare practitioner to become active. Many state organizations have Web sites to educate the public. The National Health Freedom Coalition at www.nationalhealthfreedom.org and CAMA at www.camaweb.org have links to these state associations. Set your intent towards passage of freedom legislation; pray. Find out who your State legislators are, call them, introduce yourself and let them know you support freedom legislation. Remember the saying "Freedom isn't free." You may actually have to DO something. Our brave military is forever engaged in dangerous missions to protect our freedom from the "outside." Let's work on the home front to protect our freedom within. If not you, then who?

Freedom Associations Throughout the United States

National Health Freedom Action
www.nationalhealthfreedom.com

California Health Freedom Coalition
www.californiahealthfreedom.org

Florida Health Freedom Action
www.floridahealthfreedom.org
305 668 2800

Georgia Complementary and Alternative Medicine Association
www.camaweb.org
404 284 7592

New Jersey Natural Health Coalition
www.njnhc.org
973 486 8073

New York Natural Health Project
www.NYNaturalhealthproject.org
212 946 4456

Oklahoma Health Freedom Network
http://www.oklahomahealthfreedom.org

Coalition for Natural Health
www.naturalhealth.org

Minnesota Natural Health Coalition
www.minnesotanaturalhealth.org
651 688 6515

Health Freedom Massachusetts
www.healthfreedommassachusetts.org
617 731 5510

Set My Spirit Free

As consumers and practitioners of alternative and complementary medicine, we place great importance on the integration of body, mind, and spirit. We understand their interconnection and dependence on each other. Or do we?

Let's view the field of CAM (Complementary/Alternative Medicine) from a wholistic perspective, as we would a patient – body, mind, and spirit. How would we evaluate and treat this "patient?"

Let me share my perspective on the status of the CAM body in Georgia; perhaps it is similar to your state.

I would observe that the body is weak but growing stronger. It is broken and disjointed. Imagine that the arms are hypnotherapists, the legs are naturopaths, the feet are homeopaths ... you get the picture. Now, when the arms felt threatened with the introduction of the mental health therapist legislation last session, were the feet and legs and other body parts there to support them? Did they view the body as a whole, that all parts of the body were dependent on each other? In mass I didn't see it. But I saw it more than in prior years. The body is getting stronger.

Imagine that the acupuncturists in the State of Georgia are the white blood cells of the body. The NCCAOM-credentialed acupuncturists are the neutrophils, the non-credentialed acupuncturists are the lymphocytes. Both are important, both know how to do their job, both have competent, effective members among them, both have defective members among them – just like real white cells. White cells are there to protect the body from invaders. In the presence of an invader, they multiply, seek and destroy the intruder. When HB 814, which placed non-MD acupuncturists under the total control of the Medical Board, was pushed forward by the Medical Association of Georgia (MAG), did the white blood cells rally together to put the invader in check? No. Instead, some of the neutrophils bonded with the invader instead of joining with the rest of the cells. Ever hear of the strategy of "divide and conquer?" It often works. The body was dealt a severe blow but the spirit was damaged even more. It was not simply ignoring the other body members as in the case of the hypnotherapists, but a rejection of their value and worth.

But as in the real body, there will always be renegade cells. And as in the real body, this body is resilient and will recover if the body is kept strong.

Do we understand how the body must work together in synchrony to make it strong and healthy? I think we're learning and I pray we'll learn enough - soon enough.

And how is CAM's mind faring?

The CAM mind is becoming more and more enlightened and of course much more enlightened than the non-CAM mind. But just as in the real body, a large portion of the mind (brain) is on vacation. Sometimes the CAM mind doesn't think, but simply reacts; it believes what it hears in the media and the propaganda of so-called experts. It acts on emotions instead of examining the facts. But the CAM mind is becoming more aware of the advantages of CAM as well as the advantages and value of allopathic medicine. It's beginning to explore the big picture instead of looking with a narrow focus. Quality wholistic healthcare is not a "them" versus "us;" it's a "we" proposition. The mind is becoming more willing to take an active role in its healthcare. The mind is starting to question the wisdom of medicating symptoms while ignoring the underlying cause of disease. Practitioners are learning more about CAM therapies outside their expertise. They're contributing to research and the education of others. They are beginning to understand the politics of medicine and the politics of politics. The CAM mind is becoming contemplating, questioning, thinking, analyzing.

So the body is weak but getting stronger. The mind is developing nicely.

And what of CAM's spirit?

I submit that CAM's spirit is constrained. The spirit of CAM is bound but fighting to be free. The pharmaceutical cartel and the medical establishment are working to keep it bound. Lest I be misunderstood, I am not talking about the individual pharmacist, drug representative, or medical doctor. I am talking of their powerhouse, their bureaucracy, their policy-makers. Just as it was not the people of Enron, Arthur Anderson, or WorldCom that called the shots of deception, it is not the majority of individuals in mainstream healthcare but the establishment that seeks to suppress the spirit of CAM.

Turf protection is the name of the game. Control and money are the prizes. Legislation is introduced or killed by those in power to stay in power, to restrict competition and to impede free choice for both the consumer and the practitioner. It is done under the guise of protecting the public. Allopathic medicine is often cited as the third leading cause of death. Should not their protecting-the-public work be focused on correcting allopathic medicine's shortcoming instead of restricting access to benign but effective therapies such as hypnotherapy, homeopathy, herbs, and acupuncture? The World Health Organization ranked the US 37th in healthcare quality. Most people accept that competition, increases quality and monopolies decrease quality. So why are we promoting monopolization of healthcare?

The spirit of CAM must be free and unleashed in order for CAM practitioners to fully practice and for CAM consumers to fully benefit from their gifts of healing. Can practitioners become all that they can be while continually looking over their shoulder? Can they function at their full capability while measuring every word that they speak? Wondering each day if they will receive their cease and desist order or be charged with the practice of medicine? Can consumers give all their attention to healing when they have a concern for their healthcare partner's safety and livelihood? Can consumers have a wide range of practitioners and modalities to choose from when many are practicing underground or advertise only by word of mouth? How can we have a healthy CAM patient when its spirit is oppressed?

And how can we free our spirit? We must practice what we preach, follow the advice we give our clients. Do we not tell them to take responsibility for their own body, to be proactive, to practice prevention? To not turn their body, mind, and spirit over to someone else to take care of.

Each part of our body needs to be cognizant and caring of the other body parts. We need to be whole, undivided, united, organized. Each is of equal importance, including allopathic practitioners supportive of unlicensed CAM practitioners and freedom of access. The CAM body must be kept strong to resist that which has intent to destroy or control it. We must practice preventive medicine, creating a healthy host, a healthy terrain – contributing to a strong, resistant organism.

Our mind must be sharp and knowledgeable. The time to find out about the legislative process is not when a restrictive bill is on the

Governor's desk for signature. Preventive medicine would have us learning about how to use the legislative process to prevent a bill from ever reaching the Governor's desk. And with it comes a peaceful mind. It's that *unknown* that is so unsettling. A sharp mind that knows the facts is not easily swayed by opinions and misinformation. Ignorance however acts on impulse and emotion and allows us to be manipulated. We must be healthy in body and mind to usher in a healthy spirit.

Let's practice preventive wholistic medicine for our own CAM body, mind, and spirit. Let's become informed so that we are less likely to be misled or manipulated. Let's unite so we can have a strong, healthy body to resist disease and possible death. Let's be whole. It will set our spirit free.

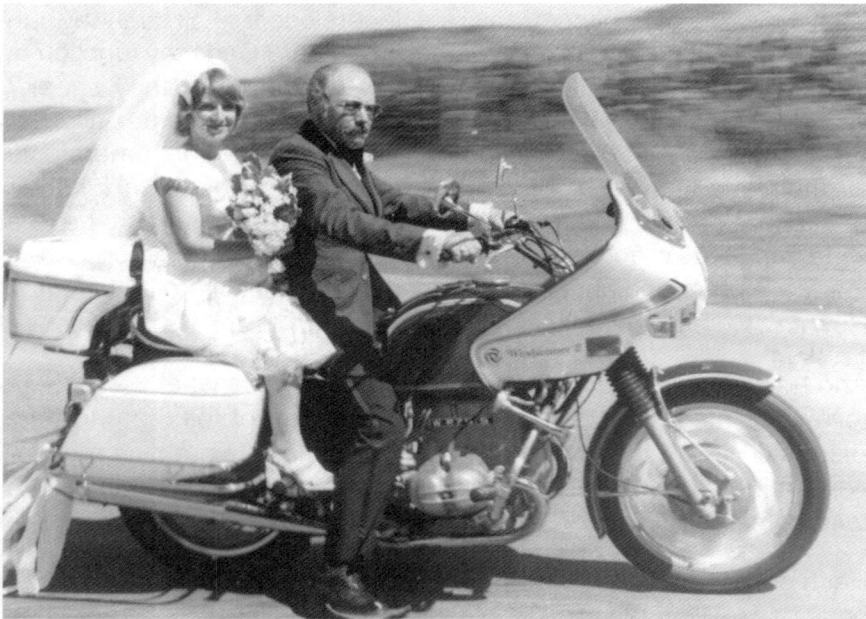

Set My Spirit Free

Leaving the church for our honeymoon.

INDEX OF PEOPLE

INDEX OF PEOPLE